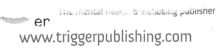

the mental health & wellbeing publisher

er

www.triggerpublishing.com

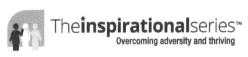

The**inspirational**series™
Overcoming adversity and thriving

Bring Me to Light
EMBRACING MY BIPOLAR AND SOCIAL ANXIETY
By Eleanor Segall

We are proud to introduce The**inspirational**series™. Part of the Trigger family of innovative mental health books, The**inspirational**series™ tells the stories of the people who have battled and beaten mental health issues. For more information visit: www.triggerpublishing.com

THE AUTHOR

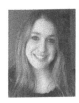

Eleanor Segall MA (hons) is journalist, mental health blog has a BA (hons) in English Lite Goldsmiths and a master's in Royal Central. She has lived w disorders since her diagnosis at

D1638940

Her mission is to increase understanding and end the stigma around mental illness.

Eleanor blogs for mental health charities such as Time to Change, Mind and SANE, and has written for publications including Metro.co.uk, The Telegraph, Glamour, Happiful Magazine, and Happiful.com. Her own blog, *Be Ur Own Light*, was recently listed as one of the top 10 UK mental health blogs by Vuelio. Eleanor is a frequent radio guest-speaker on mental health, and has recorded several podcasts. Additionally, she volunteers with the London charity Jami (Jewish Association of Mental Illness). She is a firm believer in hope, healing, talking and recovery.

First published in Great Britain 2019 by Trigger Publishing

This edition published 2019

The Foundation Centre
Navigation House, 48 Millgate, Newark
Nottinghamshire NG24 4TS UK

www.triggerpublishing.com

British Library Cataloguing in Publication Data

A CIP catalogue record for this book is available upon request
from the British Library

ISBN: 978-1-78956-036-7

This book is also available in the following e-book formats:

MOBI: 978-1-78956-039-8
ePUB: 978-1-78956-037-4

Cover design and typeset by Fusion Graphic Design Ltd

Printed and bound in Great Britain by Clays Ltd, Elcograf S.p.A

Paper from responsible sources

Eleanor's writing is insightful, honest and offers so much to those who read it. I felt like I was there beside her! She is an amazing individual.

Hope Virgo, founder of the #DumpTheScales campaign and author of *Stand Tall Little Girl*

Bring Me to Light had me gripped from page one. This is a tale of survival that everyone should read. This will shed a light on such an important topic for so many people.

Fiona Thomas, author of *Depression in a Digital Age*

Eleanor delivers a heart-breaking yet wonderful story demonstrating how sheer determination conquers all!

Karen Manton, author of *Searching for Brighter Days*

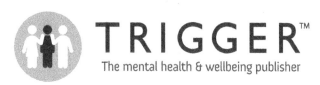

TRIGGER™
The mental health & wellbeing publisher

www.triggerpublishing.com

Thank you for purchasing this book.
You are making an incredible difference.

Proceeds from all Trigger books go directly to
The Shaw Mind Foundation, a global charity that focuses
entirely on mental health. To find out more about
The Shaw Mind Foundation visit,
www.shawmindfoundation.org

MISSION STATEMENT

*Our goal is to make help and support available for every
single person in society, from all walks of life.
We will never stop offering hope. These are our promises.*

Trigger and The Shaw Mind Foundation

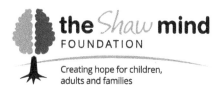

the *Shaw* mind
FOUNDATION
Creating hope for children,
adults and families

A NOTE FROM THE SERIES EDITOR

The Inspirational range from Trigger brings you genuine stories about our authors' experiences with mental health problems.

Some of the stories in our Inspirational range will move you to tears. Some will make you laugh. Some will make you feel angry, or surprised, or uplifted. Hopefully they will all change the way you see mental health problems.

These are stories we can all relate to and engage with. Stories of people experiencing mental health difficulties and finding their own ways to overcome them with dignity, humour, perseverance and spirit.

Eleanor's story is one of perseverance through difficulties with mental illness, and one that brings the realities of living with social anxiety and bipolar I disorder into sharp relief. She writes candidly about how her hospitalisation had a lasting effect on her recovery, and of how therapy and friendship were key to her wellbeing. Eleanor provides unique insight into what it is like to live with severe mental illness as a child, something that is frequently stigmatised and misunderstood. Her powerful journey of faith and purpose will inspire so many people, and show you that whatever the lowest point in your life, you can rise from it higher than ever before.

This is our Inspirational range. These are our stories. We hope you enjoy them. And most of all, we hope that they will educate and inspire you. That's what this range is all about.

Lauren Callaghan,
Co-founder and Lead Consultant Psychologist at Trigger

For my cousin Jessica z'l, a bright light that went out too soon.
To Grandpa Harry and all my family for their ongoing support.
To Rob, for giving me the confidence to share this
with the world.

This book contains reference to self-harm and suicidal thoughts.

Disclaimer: Some names and identifying details have been changed to protect the privacy of individuals.

Trigger encourages diversity and different viewpoints, and is dedicated to telling genuine stories of people's experiences of mental health issues. However, all views, thoughts, and opinions expressed in this book are the author's own, and are not necessarily representative of Trigger as an organisation.

PROLOGUE

'Welcome to the Mind Media Awards,' said Stephen Fry, reading from his Autocue and addressing the audience.

In the sixth row back from the stage, I listened intently, in disbelief that I had been invited to attend such a prestigious event.

'We are so excited to have the best of our media stars – who battle the stigma against mental health – here with us tonight,' Stephen continued. 'We have journalists, producers, writers, actors, bloggers, radio presenters, vloggers, podcasters, digital champions, TV presenters, screenwriters and filmmakers here, as well as those who have shared their mental health stories in documentaries. These awards celebrate our UK mental health advocates and awareness in the media.'

It was November 2018 and here I was, at my first ever Mind Media Awards at the Queen Elizabeth Hall in London's Southbank Centre. I was beaming, feeling fabulous in my floor-length black and gold floral embroidered dress. My dad was sitting next to me, looking smart in black suit trousers and a shirt. It meant so much that he was there with me, after all we had struggled through during our joint experiences with bipolar disorder.

In front of me, in a red sequinned dress, sat writer and journalist Bryony Gordon. I was in awe; she was a personal hero of mine, blowing me away with her honesty about her OCD and addictions. Sitting in front of her were the *Loose Women* team – including Stacey Solomon – who were presenting an award later that night; they'd often championed mental health on their show. A quick glance to my left revealed Dame Kelly Holmes, athlete and mental health advocate, and Fearne Cotton, who was seated nearby. Talented journalist Hannah Jane Parkinson of the *Guardian* – who would go on to win her award that night – also caught my eye. I knew that elsewhere in the room, actor Shayne Ward was anticipating a win for his portrayal of Aidan Connor in *Coronation Street*, who dies by suicide in the soap.

I wasn't shortlisted for an award that night, but I had been invited as a "highly commended" journalist and mental health blogger. I'd been involved in the industry for a while, writing articles in print and online on mental health topics for Mind, Metro.co.uk, *Happiful* and *Glamour* (to name a few) and writing about my own story on my blog, *Be Ur Own Light*.

'We know that media reports can have a huge impact on people's mental health, prompting them to start conversations, seek help and support each other,' says Mind, the mental health charity, on their website. 'That's why we hold the Mind Media Awards every year, to recognise and celebrate the best possible representations of mental health across TV, radio, print and online.'

Before I arrived, I'd felt pumped with adrenaline and apprehension. Yes, I was excited to be there, but I was also anxious, scared of being around so many people on such a big occasion. However, because I wasn't shortlisted, I knew I wouldn't be called up on stage. And I also knew I would regret it if I didn't go. So, after combatting my fear through a series of breathing exercises and distraction techniques, I'd found a strength I didn't know I had. That strength allowed me to fight through my social anxiety, and my dad and I set off for the Tube together.

Queen Elizabeth Hall was surrounded by twinkling Christmas fairy lights that night. In the queue to get in, my father and I got chatting to a young man who had been shortlisted for writing about mental health at university and helping fellow students through a programme there. He and his family were so down-to-earth, yet I found him incredibly inspiring. I had the opportunity to meet Katie Conibear, a shortlisted fellow blogger with lived experience of mental ill-health, and Anneli Roberts, an advocate, blogger and Twitter friend. And later, at the drinks reception, I came across Yvette Caster and Ellen Scott, my editors at Metro. co.uk. They'd been shortlisted for an award for their brilliant podcast, *Mentally Yours*. Yvette – ever so witty and kind – has bipolar disorder just like me, and has gone on to have a successful career in journalism. She'd been the first person to commission me, so I couldn't help but give her a big hug and thank her for all her help.

This was why I had come tonight: I was in my element, rubbing shoulders with those I admire most within the industry. It was so wonderful to meet these people in person; what an honour to see so much talent all in one room, all with a shared goal: to break the stigma around mental health.

It was a moving, uplifting evening. The most touching speech came from footballer Clarke Carlisle, who had gone missing very publicly due to severe depression, but had found recovery and support. Clarke told his story alongside his wife Carrie, and their passion for breaking stigma shone through, at which point they both received a standing ovation from the audience.

It was incredible to think that just four years earlier, I had been sectioned in hospital, confined to a ward, suffering a manic episode following a bout of suicidal depression. If you had told me then that four years later, I would be working as a freelance journalist for national publications and attending awards ceremonies with my heroes – sitting feet away from Stephen Fry, to boot – I would have laughed at you.

Happiful (UK mental health magazine) sponsored a chill-out zone at the drinks reception that night, and they'd put some of their issues out on the tables for people to read. What a special feeling – *my* articles were in there, and it was wonderful to know that I was making a small difference to this community.

Pointing the magazine out to my dad, who had spent years with an undiagnosed illness, never speaking about his mental health issues, made me swell up with pride. I thought about the journey he had been on, and how all of this was helping him and my family heal too.

It was the confirmation I needed: sharing my own story and writing about mental health *was* the right thing to do.

CHAPTER 1

VISITING THE PAST

In February 2018, Dad and I visited Iași, Romania, the snow-covered hometown of our ancestors.

This trip was incredibly meaningful for me and my father; our family were once involved in the now-defunct Yiddish theatre there, and some are buried in the Jewish cemetery. Yet despite its breathtaking beauty, this place would always be tainted for us, its beautiful buildings and landscape haunted by its brutal past.

Once a grand cultural hub, the Jewish community in Iași is now very small, numbering only a couple of hundred. In some of its darkest hours, many Jews were shot, killed, or piled onto trains and taken to death camps. So many Eastern European (Ashkenazi) and Sephardic European Jews lost relatives in the Holocaust, and likewise, this horrific historical tragedy had a devastating impact on both sides of my family.

Generations ago, my paternal great-grandfather Leon Segal had moved to London from Iași as a refugee, fleeing persecution in mainland Europe. Leon had no money and spoke no English when he arrived in London, but he had a strong work ethic. He worked his way up in the East London markets and went on to found a successful jewellery business in the city. It was here that he met my great-grandma, Pauline, a woman of Jewish-Romanian descent whose family had migrated from Paris to the

UK. Together they had my grandfather Carol Segal (in Eastern Europe, Carol is a man's name; he was named after King Carol of Romania), who went on to marry my grandmother Norma.

As it turned out, though, it didn't end happily for everyone in Leon's family. As we found out through Yad Vashem Holocaust Remembrance Center's online directory, Leon's sister, Olga Segal Fisher, her husband and their teenage daughters were taken from their home in 1941 and murdered in the Kishinev Ghetto (in present-day Moldova) – just for being Jewish. We don't have a grave for them, but we light a memorial candle for them every year.

Things were just as chaotic and dangerous for my mother's side of the family. My maternal great-great-grandparents moved to the UK in the 1800s to escape the Eastern European anti-Jewish pogroms (an organised massacre of a particular group). My great-grandma on my mother's side, Rosie, was born in London after their arrival from Poland. She went on to marry my great-grandpa, Sydney, who was Russian and had fled persecution as a child to come to the UK. They had my grandma Doreen in 1931.

Doreen's future husband, my grandfather Harry, was born "Hermann" Lorber in Germany in 1926. His mum, my great-grandma Sabina, fled Poland as a teenager and settled in Berlin in the 1920s, where she met my great-grandfather, Shimon. Unfortunately, they could not have foreseen what was to come for Germany's Jews.

In 1933, Hitler came to power. The Nazi regime brought with it the Nuremberg Laws, which prohibited Jews from many aspects of public life and stripped away their rights. Grandpa Harry, then aged seven, had to move to a special Jewish school. His parents, Sabina and Shimon, owned a hat-making business in Stralsund, a small coastal town in Germany, and a Nazi soldier was billeted outside their shop to prohibit people from entering. The business folded and, as times got tougher, so did the relationship. Sabina and Shimon divorced, and Sabina moved back to Berlin with my grandpa. To be a single Jewish mother trying to support yourself in Nazi Germany was no mean feat! Money and food were scarce, and it was so stressful that Sabina had a breakdown, but she eventually recovered.

Grandpa Harry remembers the 1936 Olympics and seeing Hitler on a screen outside the stadium. He was already learning in a segregated Jewish school in the Berlin synagogue and having to leave school early, so as not to incur the wrath of local anti-Semites who wanted to harm the Jewish children.

Things seemed bleak for the family when Grandpa Harry was a child. Jews knew they had to get out wherever they could, to avoid persecution and potential death. Sabina applied for visas to countries that were sympathetic to Jews, such as China. In fact, Shanghai was where Shimon ended up – he survived the war that way before making his way to Israel. At the time, countries were closing their doors to Jews and had quotas to count their numbers, but luckily, Sabina had a cousin in London who could vouch for her.

My Grandpa Harry believes that they were given a "mother and child" work visa to England by the undercover British agent, Major Frank Foley. Major Foley saved thousands of Jewish lives from his post at the Berlin Embassy Passport Office and is recognised as a righteous gentile. He realised the terrible situation that Sabina was in as a single mother with no relatives, and his benevolent act of kindness saved my family from death. Sabina was given work as a domestic cleaner, and in 1939, a few months before the start of the war, she and Grandpa Harry managed to gain passage on one of the last boats out of Germany with their visas and possessions. Sabina had stuffed her special gold necklace with Hebrew lettering into her shoe to hide it from the Nazis. My mum, her granddaughter, wears this important necklace every day.

Sabina and Harry arrived in England and settled in Cricklewood, where they were helped by the local Jewish community. Sabina later remarried, but never forgot the horrors she had lived through.

It was amazing that Grandpa and his mother got out of such a perilous situation, especially since there was such tragedy elsewhere in the family. There is a photo of Grandpa Harry's cousin holding a doll, playing outside their home in Poland in the early 1930s. They were later taken to Auschwitz and killed. Very few of his relatives survived. In the 1990s, my grandparents Harry and Doreen were shopping in a homeware store in Watford, and on the front of one of the photo albums in the shop was this photo. My grandpa broke down in tears when he saw it and recognised his cousin. We believe it was stolen by the Nazis, after which it found its way to a Danish auction house, whose staff then supplied the photo album makers with it. The auction house was not aware of the Nazi theft. It truly was a miracle that he found it just as he was celebrating his grandson's bar mitzvah.

Grandpa Harry learnt English as he grew up, becoming a British citizen and having his bar mitzvah here. He went on to serve in the British armed forces during the Second World War and was an ambulance driver in Cyprus in 1945. Miraculously, he met his cousin Bertha at a hospital in Nicosia, where they hugged and cried when she showed him the tattoo on her arm. She had survived Auschwitz and made her way to Cyprus to work as a nurse.

In 2018, the UK recognised the important work of Major Foley by unveiling a statue of him at a ceremony in his hometown of Stourbridge, attended by Prince William. Sadly, we couldn't go because of a clash with a Jewish festival, but I submitted Grandpa's story of memorial and he got an invite from the Houses of Parliament to see the statue unveiled at the ceremony. It was a very proud moment for him.

It is a true miracle, then, that my parents – Simone and Mike – even made it into the world. I exist because a family of proud, Eastern European Jewish refugees and British Jews battled against the odds to stay true to their roots and *survive*.

For this reason, our faith – and all the heritage that comes with it – is hugely important to me; it has informed my life and identity to this day.

CHAPTER 2

DISCOVERING DRAMA

Thankfully It was a happier story for my parents, Simone and Mike, who met at a mutual friend's birthday party when she was nineteen and he was twenty-four. They dated for a couple of years before getting engaged and then married three years later, in October 1983.

It was a warm summer's day in 1988 when my mum gave birth to me at Watford General Hospital, gripping my dad's hand so tightly that it nearly broke. It was a difficult delivery; the cord was wrapped around my neck so I could have stopped breathing. Luckily, though, the midwives acted quickly, and I was born healthy and well on 1st July.

Most importantly, I was born into a family that made me feel safe, loved and supported. Mum and Dad were delighted to become parents, so I was spoilt by the whole family, especially since I was the first grandchild on my dad's side and the first granddaughter on my mum's.

My younger sister Chantal and I had such an idyllic childhood. With our birthdays only a week apart, we often had joint parties and were given presents around the same time. Chantal was – and still is – my best friend, a beautiful girl with red, curly hair and a strong-willed, independent spirit. We loved to play together, two girly girls having fun with Polly Pockets, My Little Ponies and, of course, dolls – especially Barbies. We rode our bikes in the street, played games and formed secret clubs with our next-door-neighbours' children. We dug in the earth for worms and imagined digging through to Australia. In the summer, we ran under the sprinkler in the garden in our swimsuits and had water fights with our friends. We'd get completely soaked, filling the bath with bits of grass afterwards.

We were close to our grandparents growing up; Grandma Doreen and Grandpa Harry lived just down the road in Bushey, so we'd pop in to see them after school. We spent a lot of time picking blackberries with them in the country lane for Doreen's jams or pies, dark purple juice squirting everywhere – not good if we were wearing white! Other times we'd pick apples with our cousins in Grandma Norma's garden, prodding them with brooms as we were so small, and taking them home for Mum to make stewed apple or crumbles.

We would go to the children's service at synagogue every Saturday, the Jewish Sabbath, where we would see our friends, sing songs and pray (as well as eat lots of delicious food). On Sundays, we attended Sunday school to learn how to read Hebrew and find out more about our Jewish heritage.

And yet – despite all this happiness and fun – I was always a nervous child. I experienced separation anxiety at the tiny age of four, when I started primary school. I was so upset at leaving my mum and daunted at the prospect of being around bigger children in the lunch room that I was physically sick and ended up in the nurse's office.

It didn't stop there; this continued to happen for the whole of the first term! It drove my mum to distraction, as she had to come and pick me up each day and speak with my teachers about how to make it easier for me to settle in. Eventually, with help from my very kind teacher, I was able to learn to relax and eat lunch – first with her, then with my friends.

Admittedly, it particularly helped that my oldest friend, Francesca, was at school with me. Francesca and I have always been friends, and some of my happiest childhood memories involve me, Chantal, Fran and her brother, Alexander, eating pizza and chips at my house and attending Sunday school. Making friends and getting used to the routine meant that life got better, and thankfully it turned out that I loved learning.

Chantal and I did a lot of after-school activities such as Brownies, ballet, and swimming lessons. Our teacher, Cindy, was a fantastic woman who ensured we always had a good time – so much so that we carried on swimming for about a decade. Ultimately, though, I swapped swimming for drama, and I still clearly remember the day I decided that I was going to be a theatre actress. I was in Year 6 at school, and one of the other girls, Melanie, was starring as one of the orphans in a West End production of *Annie*. At break time, she showed us the song and dance routine to 'You're Never Fully Dressed Without a Smile'. To this day, I can probably sing most of the lyrics to that song in an East Coast American accent.

As Melanie sang. And as she continued to sing, I was enthralled. I went on to learn the routine with her, and something about the light-heartedness and joy of acting touched my heart. Yes, I was shy, but maybe this was the answer. Maybe if I became another character, with their own layers and complexities, people might love my performances? This realisation gave me a gift – the ability to perform on stage.

So, I asked Melanie if she knew about any local drama classes and where she was signed up. She told me she was part of a theatrical agency that had got her the part in *Annie*. There were local classes at the Margaret Howard Theatre School in Bushey, where we lived. At that time, the school had a few other bases across Hertfordshire and they taught acting and London Academy of Dramatic Art (LAMDA) exams, as well as dance classes and singing lessons. Seeing as I had two left feet coordination-wise, I decided to go with what I felt was my strength and went along to my first drama class a few weeks later.

Meeting for drama classes in a church hall with other children of the same age, we read poems, learnt how to read with expression and were trained to project our voices. We did mime and practised the art of improvisation, which is where you do a spontaneous performance with another actor or actors. Our teacher, Nikki, was an actor herself, and had starred as an extra on *EastEnders* and other BBC dramas. She was brilliant, encouraging me to enter LAMDA exams and get some experience performing at the Watford Pump House Theatre, where I was entered into the poetry festival and competed against other children in my category.

I was nervous and fiddling that day. With my mum sitting in the audience, I waited on the sidelines and watched the other children go up and perform one by one. Soon, it was my turn, and I was on edge.

I found a confidence I didn't know I had. I'd rehearsed the poem over and over again, and I could see it in my mind's eye. I just knew I could do it! I stood on the darkened stage and recited my poem, *Red* (complete with hand actions), to a panel of scary-looking judges. Although I didn't win in my category – I was up against some seasoned performers – I still got a merit certificate. I still treasure that certificate even now, because it's a reminder of a time when I found something that I was really good at.

Around the same time, I took LAMDA exams in sight reading (reading from an unseen book / piece of prose to an examiner) and mime. Mime is using bodily gestures and no sound to create a scene. The exam was a group piece, and Chantal took part in it with me (she had joined me in drama class by then). I was so proud of my LAMDA medals and kept them in a special drawer.

I stopped going to the theatre classes when I was about thirteen, but continued acting and performing throughout school. Drama was my passion and my escape and it helped build my confidence. It was certainly needed around this time for me, as there was a lot going on at home ...

CHAPTER 3

WITNESSING DAD'S MENTAL ILLNESS

I was seven years old when Dad's illness got really bad.

I'm lucky that my childhood was so wonderful, but it wasn't perfect. When I was a toddler Dad became ill with depression – although he wasn't yet officially diagnosed – and suffered from anxiety and panic attacks. He had been unwell for a while, but it got really bad the older I became, and eventually he had to stop working. Mum became the main breadwinner for the family. How hard must that have been for her? She was so young, but she now had sole responsibility for us all, taking on extra shifts in her job as an NHS podiatrist (foot doctor) and doing more private work in order to get by. She sheltered me and Chantal from it all and we spent a lot of time being looked after by my grandparents after school.

Dad went to his GP and explained his symptoms. He had to ask my grandma to drive him there and he could hardly speak during his appointment. He was prescribed Valium instead of antidepressants, and he stayed on it for nine years – but it didn't help. Dad believes that if he had been prescribed the right medication, he wouldn't have had any future episodes, but back then, no one suspected it was bipolar or a depressive disorder.

He collapsed during one particularly debilitating episode and had to spend some time in hospital. He did all he could to get well, but I know it was exceptionally difficult for him. I was so young back then that I wasn't fully aware of what was happening, but I've asked Dad. He said,

The illness started in 1991, when Eleanor was three years old. I also had panic attacks when Eleanor was four and Chantal was two. I wouldn't be diagnosed with bipolar disorder until the year 2000.

The night before my major panic attack, I had been talking to a friend who'd suffered a mild heart attack, and he described the symptoms to me over the phone. The next day was a very hot summer's day, and I had been in a meeting in a glass-roofed conservatory, without anything to drink besides a glass of orange juice. I jumped in the car to see a client for a meeting, and on entering his shop, which was airless and hot, I started to experience pains both in my chest and running up and down my left arm – the same symptoms my friend had described.

The reality was that I was about to faint from the heat and dehydration, but because I had never fainted before, I thought I was suffering a heart attack.

I went into the shop next door because they had a bench, and I asked if I could lie down on it while they called for an ambulance. When the ambulance arrived, the paramedics asked me what pains I was experiencing. They decided I needed oxygen, so they took me directly to the Royal Free Hospital in Hampstead. By the time I arrived, I couldn't feel my legs and I had severe pains in my chest and arms.

I was immediately given an electrocardiogram test (ECG), which proved that there was no problem with my heart – I was actually hyperventilating through my anxiety attack, which was exacerbated by them giving me extra oxygen. Essentially, I was taking in too much oxygen to the brain. The diagnosis was that I had experienced a severe panic attack based on the belief in my mind.

My wife and daughters arrived at the hospital just as the medical staff were completing the ECG. I was told to take the rest of the day off and then go back to work the next day. I don't remember being on medication for anxiety at this point or being given mental health support. They still hadn't diagnosed the bipolar disorder.

I was fine until a week later, when I experienced another overwhelming panic attack in the high street. I had the same chest and arm pains along with hyperventilation, which caused me to collapse in the street – but I didn't lose consciousness. I was overwhelmed and paralysed by fear, not knowing what was happening to my body. It felt incredibly real. I was convinced that blood was pouring out of my ears – even though it was a delusion of the mind, I could feel the "blood" trickling down.

I managed to stand up and get back to the office block where I worked, but I was still mid-panic attack. I got to the car park and collapsed to the floor again. I was unable to do anything until I was found by one of the secretaries. They called my mother, who worked nearby, and I was driven to her flat. I stayed in bed for two days while the symptoms gradually abated.

I then had six months of cognitive behavioural therapy (CBT) with an excellent counsellor to help me deal with the thought patterns. It was a very hard six months. I would sit in meetings with part of my brain telling me that I was having a heart attack, part of it utilising the CBT to ask 'Where is the evidence?' and dealing with the negative thoughts, while yet another part of the brain kept me having normal conversations with my colleagues. It was exhausting! Sometimes I would get so stressed I would have to leave meetings and sit in the park for a bit.

I had another panic attack near Baker Street, and had to sit on the pavement and focus on my breathing for a while. I felt stronger and able to deal with it due to the CBT and consistent therapy, but it took a while. My way of dealing with it was to block out the world by wearing dark glasses and a baseball cap and listening to music.

During those nine years in which I went undiagnosed, I experienced three manic episodes, each followed by a depressive one. Over time, each manic episode and each depressive episode got progressively worse.

In my first manic episode, my mood was always elevated. I would stay out late, going to nightclubs without my wife and spending more money than usual – all of which is typical of mania. I felt wonderful, like I could do anything, and I could not understand why people around me didn't feel the same way. But then, suddenly, it was like I'd fallen off a cliff. Like night follows day, the chemicals in my brain threw me into a deep depression overnight.

My first depressive episode (which happened in 1993) lasted three months. I couldn't work and I didn't want to see anyone or leave the house; I just wanted to curl up under the covers and stay there. I felt safe in bed, as though I was protected from the world, and didn't see the point in getting up, washed or dressed. With my wife's support, though, I was slowly able to get out of bed, go to the bathroom, and shave, despite it being draining. Eventually I felt I could walk to the newsagent, but it would take an entire day to psych myself up enough to buy a newspaper.

Eventually, I went back to work as a self-employed credit management consultant, and I stayed well for two years. Unfortunately, when Eleanor was seven and Chantal was five, I had another manic phase due to my natural brain chemistry and being unmedicated. I was mostly able to control it by ignoring the impulses to go out and spend money. However, despite the fact that this second manic episode was contained, it was immediately followed by a depression that was deeper than the first. That one lasted for four months. The depression had similar symptoms to before, although I don't remember a lot of it due to my brain protecting me. I would stay in bed all day – from nine till five – sleeping and resting. I had to stop work again and rely on help from my wife and family. I'd see my children in the evenings when I felt able to do so. Eleanor was very young, so we tried to protect her and her sister from it.

I recovered from the depression through the same slow process and engaged in further CBT, which I found helpful. I wasn't prescribed antidepressants or mood stabilisers and was never referred to a psychiatrist. However, my brain chemistry had returned to normal functioning and remained consistent for a few years. This meant that I could work again and enjoy life with my wife and young daughters – going on holiday, celebrating birthdays, and spending time with friends. For this, I consider myself lucky.

Mike Segall

*

Despite Dad being unwell, I really loved school. But as I got older, I started getting bullied by my classmates, both there and at Sunday school. It was such a sad time; though the bullying wasn't physical, I endured name calling, isolation and emotional bullying. I don't know if it was because they could sense something going on at home, because I seemed quieter and more introverted than normal, or whether I was simply an easy target for upset or frustrated children. I just don't know. My Sunday school bully is now an acquaintance of mine, so what I do know is that they were going through a hard time at home back then.

This period of my life was the first time that I really began to experience panic attacks.

In regular school, I hung out with a close group of girls, and one of them started excluding me in the playground and during group work. She used to laugh at me while telling our other friend not to talk to me, so I felt very alone. We were only seven, but she managed to make her message clear: I wasn't wanted. I was such a sensitive child and came home crying every day. I didn't enjoy learning anymore and I would feel the dread and bubbling anxiety in my stomach at the mere mention of normal school.

Sometimes I would walk into class and hear the girls giggling and whispering about me. At break times, they would call me and another friend names (silly, childish ones like "Cry Baby" or "Pig") and isolate us from their play time. They made me feel inferior, constantly sad and scared. This – on top of everything that was going on at home – sent me into a real state of panic. I used to get so worried about going to Sunday school to face my bullies there, that I would regularly cry myself into hysteria on Sunday mornings. I just couldn't cope with it at the age of seven – it was too much. It must have been horrible for my parents, especially as my dad had recently been unwell.

My parents eventually decided for me to be home-tutored for the rest of that year, at the house of a Jewish-studies teacher. It gave me a break from the constant anxiety about attending

Sunday school, and as a result I began to grow in confidence, away from all the bullies. The one-to-one attention also gave me more of an opportunity to learn about Jewish life and practice.

I felt much stronger after that year off. The bullying at regular school was stopping now because the main bully had left, so my parents decided that I would go back to Sunday school the next year, as long as I was in a different class to the child that had bullied me there.

Going back frightened me and made me apprehensive. What if I was bullied in my new class by different people? My parents had discussed with the teachers how to prevent that, but I felt like the odd one out. I was a bit geeky and I kept being picked on because I was sensitive and vulnerable. It hurt.

Feeling unsafe, I went back. And slowly I managed to settle back into the environment. I even managed to make more friends and began to thrive – Sundays didn't seem so threatening anymore. And the fact is that despite the bullying, I enjoyed school. It was a small, local, one-form-entry school that had been built in Victorian times. It was a mixed Christian primary school, but we had some brilliant teachers who were very sensitive to the fact that we couldn't always join in with that particular part of school life. I would sit through hymns in assembly and not say the word "Jesus", only taking part in the nativity play as a traveller or narrator (never Mary). We celebrated our Jewish festivals in school with the other children and my mum would bake our traditional cakes and biscuits for me to share with my classmates. I enjoyed the school discos, the Christmas post box and celebrating Chanukah – but my favourite thing was story time.

Reading has always been my escape – a magical place in which to hide and immerse myself when life around me is emotionally hard. I feel calm and safe when I'm reading, creating characters and writing, so it was no wonder that I was very strong at English. Describing scenes and escaping into stories fed my soul. It started a lifelong passion for literature and storytelling. One of my favourite books was *Charlotte's Web* by E. B. White, a story about the friendship between an intelligent spider and a pig. It is so quaintly written and so beautiful that I still enjoy it now. Our teacher read it to us chapter by chapter in Year 3, and I listened intently to every word. It gave me the freedom to switch off; I was captivated and swirled away into the story.

I was lucky to have good friends both in school and synagogue, and they all lived locally so I would see them on the weekends. We became incredibly close; they were like sisters to me. Our parents were all friends too, so we would often have play dates or celebrate festivals as families. It was reassuring to know I had such special friends in my life as we approached our teen years.

By that time, Dad had recovered from his illness and gone back to work, though he was still undiagnosed. I was simply focused on taking my Year 6 SATs tests and, of course, the eleven-plus exams to get me into secondary school. This meant a lot of revising (who needs nonverbal reasoning anyway?) and hard work, as I sat exams for many different schools. My first choice was Watford Grammar so that I could be at school with Francesca, but I didn't get in at first because I wasn't in the catchment area! By the time I *did* get in, in the January, I was already settled at my new secondary school.

My parents encouraged me to sit exams for good state schools, but also two Jewish schools – the Jewish Free School (JFS) and Immanuel College. JFS was (and still is) a really big school with about 2,000 pupils. I got a place, but because it was so big, I didn't really take to it when I visited. I was still a shy, nervous child, and so when I got a place at Immanuel College – which was a much smaller school and two minutes' walk away from my house – I decided to go there. My grandparents even lived directly opposite, so it seemed like fate!

I was very privileged to receive the amount of care and support I did there. It was a big decision for my parents because the school was fee-paying, but my dad's business and Mum's job were stable and it seemed like a great fit for me.

I settled in well during my first year at Immanuel College. I was still a little geeky and awkward, but I made a fast group of friends, including my second cousin, Anna, along with Katie, Hannah and Charlotte. In Jewish life, girls have their bat mitzvah (coming of age ceremony) at the age of twelve, so each weekend throughout Year 7 featured another girl's bat mitzvah. In Year 8 came all the boys' bar mitzvahs – many with even bigger parties. It was completely different to anything I had experienced at my Christian primary school.

My family and I are Orthodox, so when I was twelve, I had a joint bat mitzvah ceremony with Francesca and another girl at our synagogue. It had been a very difficult year for my family and money was tight again, but my parents did what they could do make my bar mitzvah wonderful and exciting.

The ceremony involved learning a curriculum and passing an exam on Jewish studies, then speaking about what you had learnt in the form of a sermon in front of an audience. We had practised for weeks with our teacher and could read from the paper, so it didn't feel too daunting on the day. I'd worked hard on this project; I was proud to read my sermon and talk about Jewish topics. This was my identity, my coming of age.

The rabbi gave us blessings, presenting us with special prayer books from synagogue. Afterwards, Fran had her party in a local hotel (during which I made a toast to her) and I had a few smaller parties at home with friends and family, including a disco (which were all the rage back in 2000) and a sit-down lunch with loved ones.

It was an important, memorable, fun occasion, and yet, I still found the attention – and the presents that came with it – hard. I didn't feel like I deserved it. Dad was so unwell; didn't he deserve it more?

It was only a few months before my bat mitzvah that my dad became ill again, this time with a very serious depression. I was sheltered from a lot of his emotions, but I could tell something was seriously wrong. Dad had had depression before, but this one was more serious. He was very tearful and sleeping and hiding a lot in his bedroom, pulling the duvet over his head. He couldn't work and my mum couldn't communicate easily with him. Chantal, like me, didn't understand depression either, as she was only ten years old. But she does remember that his illness affected the mood in the house. Also like me, she was constantly stressed and upset, feeling "vulnerable" and that "things weren't right". There was also a sense for us both that money was tight, and although we were children, we realised that all was not well.

One morning before school, at about half past seven, my sister and I were getting ready and putting on our uniforms, when we heard a slight commotion in the bathroom. What we didn't know was that my brilliant dad was so ill he was standing in front of the mirror, holding about eighty aspirin tablets in his hands, and contemplating taking them all. He was considering whether to take his own life.

Apparently, Mum had walked in and seen him with the tablets. Calmly, she'd asked, 'Are you going to take those?'

'No,' he'd replied.

'Please put the tablets away,' Mum had said, and Dad had dropped the medication and returned to bed. She then promptly called my aunt (who is a GP) and asked her to come and talk to him. They got my dad a referral back to see a psychiatrist urgently.

I didn't fully grasp the extent of what was happening. I was just told to take my sister to my grandparents so that we would be out of the house.

Unbeknown to him, this was a depressive episode brought on by his bipolar disorder. Some years later, as I spoke to Dad about what happened, he told me that he didn't take his own life because of his wife and children.

In 1999, I found that I was becoming unwell again, despite having a stable family home. My brain chemistry was left untreated and I had another manic episode with the same previous symptoms – an elevated mood and the urge to spend money and party. I didn't do this though; I recognised the mania immediately and was able to deal with it, with little noticeable effect to others.

However, when the third manic episode finished, I was plunged into the deepest, darkest suicidal depression that I had ever experienced. I was still going to work, but the thoughts going through my head were, 'Life is too painful and I can't deal with this anymore. I want to die.'

I was so ill that, when taking the Tube to work, I began to visualise stepping in front of the train and ending my life. On every occasion, the love of my wife and young children came into my mind and stopped me from doing it.

At other times, I would be driving my car down the motorway when I'd think about speeding up and crashing my car into a barrier. It felt very real, and I pictured it more than once. I needed relief from my pain of depression and saw no way out, no way of getting help from mental health services.

The depression lasted for five months, during which time my suicidal ideation gradually lessened. I spoke with my GP, who had noticed that despite having six major episodes of mania and depression, I had never been referred to a psychiatrist or put on mood-stabilising medication. I am thankful to them for organising a referral to a psychiatrist, Dr N.

My wife and I went to meet with Dr N at Priory Hospital North London, where Eleanor would later be treated. I was hopeful that this would help me. My wife had to supply the doctor with extra information because I couldn't remember it all and it was very painful to recount. It was this that confirmed to Dr N that my manic and depressive episodes were bipolar 1 disorder.

I felt relieved by the diagnosis. I was slowly weaned off Valium and then put on to Lithium Carbonate to stabilise my moods. I was thankful that the Lithium worked and continues to work. It is now almost twenty years later and I have not had a serious episode of mania or depression since.

Mike Segall

*

Dad was forty when he received this diagnosis. He was helped to recovery through medication (Lithium) and CBT. But no one knew that, as I entered my teen years, I would be at risk of those mental health issues myself ...

CHAPTER 4

MY FIRST LOVE

I was a teenager now, and, in Jewish law, an adult – though I certainly didn't feel like one! I was enjoying school and growing into myself slowly.

Francesca and I were still friends, but she was at a different school now, so I didn't see her as much. I missed her and that feeling of comfort she gave me, especially when I started getting teased for having a thick, curly fringe that would never stay straight and train-track braces on my teeth. By the time I was fourteen, however, I had become much more confident in myself. The braces had come off, I had grown out my fringe, I started getting periods and was becoming a woman. I felt so much better; I socialised more, having sleepovers, watching films, going to parties, having "boyfriends" (though not proper ones) and other girly activities. So far, so normal for a teenager.

I continued with drama, taking on small parts in the school plays: Shakespeare's *The Tempest*, Gogol's *Our Town*, and Arthur Miller's *The Crucible*. In *The Crucible* – a GCSE Drama play I acted in in Year 10 – I played the role of Mrs Putnam, a middle-aged woman whose children had passed away shortly after birth. The lines I had to practise were intense – they were about dead babies, after all. But interestingly, it helped my acting. It meant I had to dig deep into my emotions and imagine what it might be like to live through such a tragedy.

Drama made me happy in school, to the point that I felt positive and content at the end of Year 10. I'd enjoyed the year, visiting Strasbourg, spending time with my friends, camping in Devon with my Jewish youth group and socialising with people all over the country. I wasn't looking forward to going into final year of GCSEs in the autumn, but I knew I would face it.

I felt most free at around fourteen or fifteen years old, the year before I became unwell. Life seemed exciting and I was more carefree. That year was also the year I met someone who would impact my life for years to come.

In September 2003, I started Year 11, my final GCSE year. There was no hint of what was to come with my mental health, though it makes sense as to why it was about to change. Doctors often say that in puberty, hormones can spark mental health issues due bodily changes. I was also genetically predisposed to having issues, due to my dad having bipolar disorder.

I met Joe, my first love, in the October, at a leaving party for a friend who was going back home to live in Australia. I spent the night laughing and chatting, taking photos, getting my hair straightened with GHDs and putting on a flattering white jumper and little denim skirt.

At some point I went outside to get some air, when our friend Ben from school arrived, bringing Joe with him. We hadn't expected him to bring anyone, but instead of being annoyed, I instantly felt what can only be described as a gravitational pull towards Joe. He was tall, dark and handsome, and I wanted to know more about him.

I went inside the house and found my friends, but I was now hyper-aware that Joe was around. My every sense was attuned to him. It was just lust, but I felt this crazy urge to engage him in conversation. So when Joe went into the garden to smoke a cigarette, I decided to go out and introduce myself.

That night we started talking about our lives, discussing anything and everything. I found out that he was living with a family in North London. Unlike my parents, his were divorced and one of them had remarried. He wasn't living with them and his mum lived abroad.

I was intrigued. Joe was so charming, and I had never met anyone like him. He captivated me.

Some people drank that night, and some people didn't. But we were all carefree teenagers, enjoying life, running around in the garden and into the playing fields behind Anna's house. When our friends started going back inside the house – and only a few hours after we had met – Joe and I kissed for the first time.

And that was that. I was smitten.

It wasn't plain sailing after that. We started seeing each other, having our first date at the cinema. It didn't turn into a full relationship, though, largely because of Joe's difficult home situation. He was struggling, and being a teen is hard enough without that kind of adversity. I'm an empath, and I took his situation very much to heart. Despite our different upbringings, I felt we had a connection. I wanted to take care of him, to help him and give him the love he needed.

But I couldn't. I was becoming unwell.

My mood was getting lower and lower, and by November I was depressed. I'd begun to withdraw and became increasingly anxious and out of control. My heart would race and I would get palpitations. Perhaps it was the onset of puberty and my family's history of bipolar disorder that triggered it. I was dealing with exams, too, and putting pressure on myself to help Joe.

I cared about Joe so much, but we were too young and immature, and Joe was going through a lot. I was sensitive and vulnerable, and could barely help myself, let alone him. I just couldn't deal with any instability, and so eventually, Joe broke up with me. It was incredibly hard.

Joe knows and understands that I don't blame him at all for me becoming ill – we were children; he couldn't help what was going on in his life. It was just unlucky that all this happened while I was developing a chronic mental illness. Thankfully, we went on to be an ongoing supportive presence in each other's lives.

My school was concerned that I wasn't coping, so they told my parents that it may be a good idea to for me to see my school counsellor. She was a kindly soul, with a smiley, open face and curly hair. I don't remember a lot about our counselling sessions – we may have had three or four – but I do remember that part of our school (which was an old stately home) had a high tower and that the room was right at the top! It was a small, welcoming room and I would come and pour my heart out to the counsellor. I would often cry, terrified about the future and what was going on in my life.

My mental health was deteriorating, so my counsellor suggested that I should see a child psychiatrist. She was right; in the end, I became so ill with agitated depression that I had to take six weeks off school.

I was so frightened that I couldn't switch off. I was restless and I couldn't sleep well. My body had convinced itself that it was in danger and I was pumped with adrenaline all the time. I had never felt this way before. I was just fifteen years old and I was petrified.

Our GP, who had known me since I was a baby and knew about my dad's bipolar disorder, came out to see me. I didn't want to be around people, but I knew I needed help and fast. When the GP arrived, my anxious thoughts were racing and I was so agitated I couldn't get my words out. It sounded like I was hiccupping because I couldn't finish my sentences. Every sense was heightened. I felt depressed, deflated, yet I was highly aware of everyone around me.

'How are you feeling?' the doctor asked, and I did my best to respond, but my mum often had to step in because I found it extremely hard to describe the state I was in. A kindly man, the doctor told us it would be best if I were referred to a psychiatrist. He prescribed me emergency medication – tranquilisers and antidepressants – which made me nervous. I had never taken them before, but I knew I needed them for my recovery.

In order to be seen quickly, my GP requested that we go to a private child psychiatrist near our home. Luckily, this was approved, and within days I was walking up the stairs in my school uniform, ready to meet my first ever psychiatrist.

'It sounds like you're in a depressive state due to stress,' he told me, prescribing me an antipsychotic called Olanzapine.

I couldn't really do much while I waited for the medicine to kick in; I felt so anxious, and my heart and thoughts were racing so quickly that I just dozed under a blanket on the couch, listening to Classic FM to try to escape from it all. The Olanzapine really helped me to get better and to find clarity, but it *did* make me put on a lot of weight. I'd always been slim, so now I was very self-conscious.

As I recovered from the depression – losing weight in the process, due to my fast teenage metabolism – I started processing what had happened. I knew I had spiralled into panic and anxiety, that I hadn't slept, and that I was exceptionally vulnerable to stress triggers. My main fear was about how I would catch up on my school work in such a key year of my education; I needed my GCSEs in order to achieve what I wanted in life.

This was a huge preoccupation for me, so school set out a plan to help. Teachers were on hand to provide support and give me extra tutoring to catch up on what I had missed. I started reading textbooks to improve my concentration, did some practice papers for my exams, and began to make notes on my subjects.

I started back at school very slowly and carefully; I was stable again but still very fragile, so even attending one lesson a day exhausted me. It took a lot of effort, and I still felt very self-conscious. Luckily, my friends were fantastic and came to visit me to provide love and support, photocopying their school books and bringing me notes. My grandparents supported my mum and dad, too. I was surrounded by get-well cards, cakes and presents. It honestly meant the world to us.

I gradually got better and felt strong enough to go back to class. I admit I was still exceptionally anxious about it – I didn't know what people would think. How would I explain my absence? Would people judge me? But thankfully, people were very wrapped up in their lives and my friends were incredible, making sure I felt safe and got to lessons again. My psychiatrist continued to monitor me, and with their help, I got through the year despite the depression.

Unfortunately, I was no longer able to take my drama GCSE, because before I'd been hospitalised, I'd became quite distressed in one of my drama lessons. A group consisting of me, my close friend Charlotte, and two boys had begun writing dialogue for a play, and I'd created a character similar to myself. The theme was domestic violence. My character was vulnerable and I'd written her so that her emotions would unravell on stage, as that was exactly how I'd felt at the time. But then I'd taken time out after six weeks of depression at home, and now that I'd returned, I was back to performing a depressed character that I'd created before I had left.

Our teacher asked us to rehearse our piece in the school theatre, which had recently been decorated with black walls. Apprehensively, I walked up the wooden steps to the small stage. I looked around at the rest of the class, who were busy performing and perfecting their pieces for the exam. My heart rate shot up immediately; my hands and face were clammy and breaking out with beads of sweat. Everything slowed down. I felt completely exposed and on show – but I knew I still had to rehearse.

Charlotte said her line, but when it was my turn to respond, I took one look at the script in my shaking hands and burst into floods of tears.

'El?' Charlotte said, concern in her blue eyes. 'Are you okay?'

I just shook my head. I couldn't speak as I was crying so much, so Charlotte went to get our drama teacher. I just wanted to hide away.

Our teacher, Mrs Endelman, a kind lady with curly brown hair and sparkly eyes, came over. She had known me for a year or so and was aware of me being unwell and off school. She took me aside gently, offered me a tissue and calmed me down, away from the rest of the class. 'Eleanor, what's wrong?' she asked.

'How can I help?'

'I don't know,' I said. 'I just can't perform today. The character I've created is making me feel really anxious and worried. I don't feel able to play her.'

'Would you like to go somewhere to calm down? Maybe Charlotte can go with you,' Mrs Endelman suggested.

Thanks to her kindness, I was able to go with Charlotte to an empty classroom and take time out from the stress and pressure I was feeling. Char calmed me down and made me smile, helping me to feel okay again, though I was incredibly embarrassed that I had cried in class. I loved this subject with all my heart, but my emotions were at breaking point. I couldn't cope with any extra stress; I especially couldn't deal with playing a character I'd created to embody how I was feeling.

I hadn't yet been diagnosed with bipolar disorder when this happened, so it took a while for me to get back to normality and stop feeling so vulnerable and scared. Since I was too unwell and anxious to perform on stage, the exam board ruled that I could not have an alternate assignment or achieve my GCSE. It really hurt; drama was my favourite thing to do and I had worked so hard on all my assessments. Being a good actress and enjoying drama was a big part of my identity, and I'd been on track to get an A*, so it was upsetting to learn that I wouldn't even get a grade. When I look back now, I realise it was total stigma – these days, I don't think they would be allowed to get away with it.

As such, my Child and Adolescent Mental Health Services (CAMHS) psychiatrist advised me not to study drama at A Level because it could trigger me again. So, as a precaution – and supported by my teachers, parents and psychiatrist – I put my love for theatre on the back burner. At least, academically.

I had always used drama to cloak myself in my imagination, where I became someone else and portrayed it on stage. Drama boosted my self-esteem because I knew that, when I was well, I could act as someone else – I didn't have to be shy, sixteen-year-old Eleanor. I could become someone twenty years older or ten years younger, with a completely different life story. Performing made me feel good too, so to have it taken away was painful. I have always loved losing myself in others stories, whether through literature or performance. I had spent hours analysing plays and writing essays for two years, and it felt like all my hard work for the subject I loved was going to waste. Not only that, but I had dreamt of being an actress on the West End since I was a child (although dancing didn't come naturally to me), so this felt like a major setback. I didn't know if I would ever get to drama school, or even get to study at university at all without this drama GCSE.

When results day came around that summer, I walked through the school gates nervously. I had been worrying all night about my exam results and didn't know what to expect. My mum and dad accompanied us as my friends and I stood there, clutching our brown envelopes. I slowly ripped mine open and looked down at the piece of paper that would determine my future.

I was overcome with joy. The results were surprisingly excellent – all A*–B. What a surprise to everyone after my six weeks of depression, my time off school with the psychiatrist and having to get better in order to even sit my exams.

I couldn't believe it. I was teary and my dad cried. We'd all been through so much to get here. Ultimately, my sheer determination that my illness wouldn't affect my results, along with the stable support of my family and school, had helped me to pass my exams.

It was a staggering achievement.

CHAPTER 5

EXPERIENCING ISRAEL

As bipolar disorder is episodic, there is a "mood cycle", where one can go from depression, to functioning, to mania, and vice versa. Over the weeks following GCSE results day, my depression cleared and my brain was functioning normally, but because I hadn't been diagnosed with bipolar disorder, the next mood change went unseen until it got particularly bad.

I was elated. I socialised a lot, feeling very happy and a little hyper, but nothing too out of the ordinary. My family just assumed it was because of my good results and my relative freedom over the summer before A Levels.

My doctor cleared me to go on a four-week tour of Israel with my youth group. Exploring their homeland with friends is a rite of passage for a lot of Jewish teenagers around the world. I couldn't wait to go, particularly as quite a few of my friends were in my tour group. I'd never been to Israel before, and I was particularly excited about seeing Jerusalem, Tel Aviv and the north of Israel. Israel is such a big part of my Jewish identity; the Old City and the Western Wall of the former Jewish temple ("The Kotel" in Hebrew) are holy to Jewish people.

As I walked through Jerusalem amongst the beautiful sandstone walls, I was in awe. Approaching the Western Wall for the first time, I became tearful. I couldn't believe I was on the site of our former temple. I prayed at the wall, joyful tears falling down my cheeks. It was a pivotal moment in my life.

Unfortunately, that entire fourteen-day trip in Israel was pivotal, for a different reason: I experienced an encounter with hypomania, a lesser manic episode.

My thoughts began to race again and I talked rapidly. I was vulnerable to being exploited by other teenagers. I was acting out of character, becoming very flirtatious and inappropriately affectionate to others. I never had full sex with anyone, but engaging in any sexual activity with guys I didn't know well was scandalous to those I was away with – sexual activity before marriage isn't allowed in Orthodox Judaism. Since the trip was being led by an Orthodox group, everyone around me was conditioned to think that we had to be "good girls" and not engage in activity beyond kissing – especially not with teenage guys we had just met. Usually, I wouldn't have done any of it at all, but the hypomania had sent my libido sky-high.

As my hypomania progressed over several days, I became more unwell and more hyperactive. This meant I would pace around and be disinhibited with others without realising, making inappropriate sexual comments and hugging people randomly. I talked manically and was a more exuberant, hyper version of myself.

All of this had effectively come out of nowhere.

It was incredibly difficult and embarrassing for me. I was ashamed of the sexualised side of me that hypomania brought out, and I was made to feel like a slut by some others who didn't fully understand my behaviour, not knowing I was ill. People spread rumours about me and some friends distanced themselves because they didn't understand what was happening to me. Teenagers can be cruel, and I cried on lots of occasions. I was just an ill teenager trying to make a good impression on my friends and peers, failing miserably due to my undiagnosed illness.

Fortunately, I had made some friends on that trip, so it wasn't all terrible. It was these friends who were so concerned that they spoke to our youth leader, who was a wonderful human being. She had so much compassion and empathy. She phoned my parents, and alarm bells immediately started ringing. They came up with a plan for my dad to fly out to come and take me back to friends of my family, before flying back to the UK to see my psychiatrist.

They didn't tell me this was happening; rather, when we were in Jerusalem one Friday before Shabbat (the Jewish Sabbath), my youth leader told me that my dad had arrived to see me. Being so hyperactive, I was overjoyed and didn't suspect that his being there was out of character. I accepted his narrative that we were going to spend Shabbat with some family friends.

I sat in the car while my dad put my pre-packed suitcases in the boot, and then we sped off.

'It's so good to see you!' I told him. 'I'm really looking forward to this.'

Dad looked at me, his face flushed from the sun, and suddenly a serious expression came over his face. 'Els,' he said. 'I'm sorry to tell you this. We've been really worried about you and your health, and so have your friends.'

I was instantly annoyed. 'Why are my friends worried?' I demanded. 'And why did they tell you?'

'It's because you aren't yourself right now,' Dad said carefully. 'We think you could be ill again, so we've decided to take you home from the trip.'

I felt a flash of anger and shock. *How can I be unwell when I am so happy? I'm having such a fun time! I'm on holiday!* I thought. Why was I being taken off a trip where I was having the time of my life?

Why me, and why now?

'Dad, I don't want to go home,' I insisted. 'I am totally fine!' Dad didn't look convinced. 'When we get there, I'm phoning Mum. I want to stay on the trip – I can't leave halfway through! It's not fair!'

I had no idea or insight that I could be manic. I hadn't yet been diagnosed, so as far as I was concerned, I was just being a happy version of myself. But that didn't matter. When I spoke to my mum, she told me I couldn't stay on the trip. I had to come home to see my doctor.

The tears came then, but so did a kind of tacit acceptance. I was going to have to fly home.

Maybe I knew subconsciously that I needed help. However angry I felt about leaving, maybe the fact that my dad had flown out to assist me and look after me meant that something was very wrong. I still felt seriously angry though, and it still took time to accept the truth – that I would have to leave Israel.

When I saw my psychiatrist, he still wasn't sure whether or not I was suffering from hypomania. He believed that the heat and the stress of the Israeli trip contributed to my disinhibition and hyper state, so prescribed me some tranquilisers and requested that I get a lot of sleep and look after myself.

But Mum had seen my dad go through periods of bipolar illness and decided she wanted to get a second opinion, so I was referred to the child and adolescent psychiatrist at the Royal Free Hospital in Hampstead, London. I got an appointment to see my new doctor in the September.

It took months for me to come down from my high state, and I was scared of what was to come. Did I just have depression and anxiety? What was the hyper behaviour? Was I really just stressed and tired? Or could it be something more sinister? I was only sixteen and had been through so much that year already.

I didn't really know what to make of life that summer, and I had no idea that the fabric of my life was going to be ripped apart again. Why was I having such a rough time? I was supposed to be having the time of my life, forming my identity. But I didn't really know who I was and that was scary. I was dealing with the trauma of bipolar episodes and not being in control of my own mind. I was frightened, my life filled with uncertainty and a confused sense of self.

And yet, despite all this, I still had to focus on starting the first year of my A Levels. I had no choice.

CHAPTER 6

GOING INTO HOSPITAL

After a month or so of getting lots of sleep and taking regular medication, I seemed to come down naturally from the high. I presented as my "normal" self, though I was a bit sad and anxious about what had happened. I was desperate to get back to some semblance of a normal teenage life – whatever that meant.

In September 2004, at the same time as I started studying for my A Levels at Sixth Form and met my new psychiatrist at the Royal Free Hospital. That meeting changed the course of my life. Although I was now stable, he wanted to monitor me, and asked me to come back and see him in a few months with an update on how I was doing. Unfortunately, by the November, I was already falling increasingly unwell.

Having bipolar disorder can be incredibly challenging sometimes. My mood was gradually becoming lower and I was incredibly vulnerable to stressful triggers. One such trigger happened after I spoke to Joe; I had seen him around over the summer and we were still in touch. It was like we couldn't be apart! Often, however, he didn't understand what was happening and what the manic phases meant for me. How could he? We were only sixteen and none of us knew what my condition actually was, so it was hard for everyone.

After a tough phone call, Joe made a comment about what was going on in his life, and it triggered fear within me. I was already starting to go into psychosis at this point, and since I hadn't had help for it, that psychosis was heightened. My thoughts became muddled and I lost touch with reality. I began to have regular panic attacks about fear triggers and I wasn't sleeping well.

This was an undiagnosed bipolar episode, and it swiftly turned my pain and panic into a depressive state and full-blown psychosis. I started having extreme panic attacks again which, for me, were terrifying. I would cry, my heart would beat very quickly, I'd hyperventilate and I would focus on scary, negative thoughts. I was in emotional pain, and I cried and screamed because I just couldn't cope with that level of anxiety. My parents didn't know what to do.

'Mum, I can't deal with this. I can't deal with these thoughts,' I sobbed, as I curled into a ball on the sofa. 'I just want to die.'

'Ellie,' Mum said calmly. 'It's okay. I'm here.'

'No, Mum!' I screamed. 'I just want to die! Go away!'

Mum looked devastated, stunned, as though I'd slapped her across the face. But she tried to remain calm, comforting me and repeating over and over again that she was there for me.

Fear tore through me. What was happening?

To make things worse, I started to experience delusions, forming false beliefs about men abusing me and my dad. Fear of danger, being hurt or being abused is common when the mind enters a psychotic state, and I was suffering. Joe never hurt or abused me but starting a relationship when I was becoming ill caused my thoughts to become confused.

That night, I feared (wrongly) that I had been sexually abused, and that I was being drugged and poisoned when my dad administered the tranquilisers that had been prescribed to me to help me calm down and sleep. I was so frightened that I actually ran out of the house and into next door's, despite Dad looking after me and trying to keep me safe.

'Help me,' I told my neighbours as they tried to calm me down. 'My family are trying to hurt me!' What they made of an unwell sixteen-year-old making such devastating and untrue claims, I have no idea. To their credit, though, they managed to calm me down and were very kind when Dad came to find me.

I was out of control. My parents phoned my psychiatrist, who could see I was suffering from an acute phase of mental illness and needed medical treatment. I told my parents that I didn't feel safe at home with my illness. I wanted to be looked after in hospital, but it was Christmas and most places were full. Through an absolute miracle, my psychiatrist found me a bed at the specialist adolescent unit at the Priory Hospital North London, not far from home.

The next thing I knew, Mum was driving me in the dark to the hospital. We drove down the long, winding gravel driveway towards this big building, the place that would be my home for the next four months. It looked like a stately hotel with its butterscotch sandstone pillars.

The admission process is a bit of a blur in my mind. All I remember is the extreme anxiety, the lack of sleep, the racing heart and adrenaline, and the disorientation caused by the psychosis, coupled with sedation once I was put on medication. I think my brain has blocked out a lot to protect me.

I was still all over the place, but still I knew that ultimately, I would get the help I desperately needed.

CHAPTER 7

ENTERING THE PRIORY

Most people know the Priory as the chain of private mental health hospitals and rehab centres for the rich and famous, but I attended the Child and Adolescent Mental Health Services unit. CAMHS is a specialist unit for the treatment of young people with a wide variety of mental illness. It prides itself on its caring and supportive attitude to its young patients and their recovery. As such, my care was solely funded by the NHS. The CAMHS unit was up a flight of stairs separate to the main hospital, which catered to adults, some of whom were on the renowned Addictions Rehab unit.

It was Christmas Eve when I entered the adolescent unit and met the nurses for the first time. I knew they were there to help me, but I was still feeling confused and frightened, as I didn't fully grasp the enormity of what was happening due to my psychosis and anxiety. I was led to my room, which, much like a hotel room, had its own bathroom, TV, wardrobe, bed, mirror and chest of drawers. My mum and the nurse helped me to unpack my bags and hang up my clothes in the wardrobe.

And then the time came for Mum to leave me there.

I cried at the thought; I hated the idea of being left here without her. What would happen next? How could I cope with meeting the other patients? It must have been gut-wrenching for

Mum to leave me, but I desperately needed the help that only the specialist unit could give me.

As a voluntary patient who had elected to go into hospital, I suppose, in theory, I could have left at any time. But I was so unwell it was likely that if I had asked to leave or attempted to abscond, I could have been sectioned for my own safety, especially since I was under eighteen and therefore there was even more of a duty of care for me.

Some of the other people on the ward were lovely – they wrote me notes and cards to say hello, told me not to be frightened, and wished me a merry Christmas. They tried to include me in their conversations and welcome me when I was feeling scared. They all knew how anxiety-provoking it was to be a teenager in hospital. Most of them had been in hospital for a while due to depression, schizophrenia, addictions, anxiety disorders, eating disorders and other mental illnesses. This meant that the ward was always lively, but at times it was a difficult and chaotic place to be. One morning, I woke up to find that I had slept through one of the other patients destroying the staff computer in anger. The patient, who had schizophrenia, had turned the computer upside down and smashed it on the floor. Despite this, though, I did make friends there and it was amazing to watch people recovering in "real time".

On the ward, we had a lounge where everyone could go and socialise and watch TV, a kitchen to make drinks and toast (our other meals were prepared downstairs), and the nurses' station, along with individual bedrooms. There was also a big room at the end where we did group therapies such as music therapy, dramatherapy, PE and exercise, along with one-to-one counselling. The Priory also had grounds with a lake, gardens where we could go with the nurses and therapists, and rooms for art therapy (which even had a kiln to make pots out of clay!). There was a kitchen where we did cookery and a school room where we tried to work and stay on top of our education.

Going to school in hospital was an experience, because the patients on the ward – and therefore students – ranged in age from eleven to eighteen. We had one small classroom on the hospital site, and one very patient teacher, Patrick, who had to teach each of us at our own level. I was hospitalised during the first year of my A Levels – for which I was studying English Literature, History, Religious Studies and French – so my fantastic teachers at Immanuel College sent me work to do. I tried my hardest to write essays, but it was a challenge when I wasn't feeling at my best. The classroom was rather noisy and some of the other patients didn't want to work; we often found people hiding in the classroom cupboard, playing guitar, while the rest of us were attempting to be studious. Schoolwork and getting off the ward gave some structure to my day, but it wasn't easy. I eventually went down a year at school to catch up. I couldn't help but be disappointed. I'd always been a good, hardworking student, and now I'd have to find a new social circle as well.

As I said before, my parents suspected I had bipolar disorder. Mum had noticed similar signs and behaviours to those of my dad, who had been diagnosed only four years earlier, despite having experienced depression and mania since he was a teenager. I kept imagining that I'd been harmed and abused, so I wouldn't let Dad see me. It must have broken his heart, even if he did know it was because I was ill. Dad had never had psychosis.

My parents and I met with my new psychiatrist in a small consulting room of the Priory. I had been hospitalised due to a mixed depressive episode, but I'd also had episodes of hypomania and psychosis that year, so, knowing my family history, the doctor diagnosed me with bipolar affective disorder, type one.

I now had a chronic mental health condition that would mean I would have to take medication for the rest of my life. There was no cure, only management of the condition.

It took time to sink in, and I didn't figure out the enormity of this – and what it would mean for my life – until I left hospital. As a teenager, you only ever want to fit in, but my illness made me stand out.

A few months into my stay, when I was getting used to my new medication and my thoughts had calmed down, my medical team decided that I should receive one-to-one counselling from a therapist on the ward. Her name was Susannah, and she was probably in her twenties. She was a dramatherapist by training, and although we didn't do drama therapy together due to my vulnerability, I felt like she was a kindred spirit. We met every week in the therapy room for chats about how I was feeling and getting on with my new diagnosis. She was an excellent therapist.

I looked forward to having a safe space and sounding board for all my worries each week. I was only sixteen and still a child in UK law, so to feel like I was being heard while going through such a difficult time was vital. It meant that I could begin to process what had happened and that I'd had a psychotic episode. Psychosis was very new to me, so we talked about recovery and how to stay well on my new medication, as well as how to look after myself. I felt an affinity with Susannah; she would listen to my fears and worries and patiently advise me on how to deal with them.

I was so thankful for Susannah's kindness, but felt a bit down about having to leave her therapy sessions once I was handed over to the community team. In all honesty, despite my focus on getting well, it took me years to properly process the delusions, anxiety and psychosis that I'd been through.

As my mind was slowly returning to normal functioning, I began to appreciate the people on the ward. The nurses in particular were great. On the days when I didn't want to get out of bed, they would slowly coax me out and help me get washed. One nurse even came into my room and helped me to apply my mascara (somehow, looking good was still important to me, even in hospital!).

When I began to get more independent again, I'd have a laugh with the staff and my friends on the ward. Sometimes, the nurses would accompany us to therapy groups, including art and cookery. One day, one of the nurses was tasked with taking a few of us to the supermarket to buy ingredients for a pasta bake for that day's cookery session. This was to help us to reintegrate and get used to the outside world again. Being out in public made me feel quite self-conscious – what if people saw me and thought I was unwell? – but I was soon put at ease. Leaving the ward was a real treat, and it was helpful to feel like a "normal" person again, integrating back into the world beyond the hospital.

I had settled into a hospital routine of breakfast, therapy group, lunch with the others, afternoon group or time reading celebrity gossip magazines (I can tell you all the gossip from 2004 – for example, Kerry Katona went into the Priory for her bipolar disorder, and Jordan and Peter Andre had fallen in love on *I'm A Celebrity!*). We also socialised in the lounge with the many people on the ward. Dinner was then at about six o'clock in the dining room where we had lunch, and afterwards, my mum would often appear and we'd go up to my room and have a chat about our days. Sometimes, Mum would run me a bath and then I would get into bed to chat with her. I was always sad when she left, but I would distract myself by watching some good reality TV. Before I knew it, it would be time for evening medication (my new mood stabiliser and antidepressants) and bed.

It took some getting used to taking medication at first. I felt like my whole life had changed. My psychiatrist told me there was currently no cure and, as it was a chronic illness, that I would be likely to be medicated for the rest of my life. How terrifying. I was so young, with my whole life ahead of me. How was I going to manage a chronic, unpredictable illness?

There is so much we don't know about the causes of bipolar disorder. Research has moved on since 2004 and doctors now know that mood-stabilising medication and antipsychotics, coupled with therapy and good support networks, can help manage the illness and keep you well. However, stressful life events and home environments can still impact on you negatively.

I was fortunate to be correctly diagnosed at such a young age and to receive outstanding care in my first hospital admission. I have met people who have been sent thousands of miles away from home without proper support. Others have been misdiagnosed or do not identify with their diagnosis. So, when I look back at my time in hospital, I'm grateful to have been near my home and to have supportive family and friends. I know not everyone is so lucky.

My school friends sent me two big cards filled with messages, which meant a lot. Mental health was much less discussed in 2004 and I had been bullied at my youth group, so I really panicked about what they thought. As things were so chaotic on the ward, staff decided it would be better for my friends not to visit, so instead they sent me photos and wrote me letters about their normal teenage lives. I missed them terribly.

As I got better, I was allowed to spend a few weeks at home on the slow lead-up to my discharge date from the unit. This was good, but at times it was challenging as my emotions were all over the place. I was angry, hurt, unsure of myself and irritated that I was being watched so closely. Mum and Dad questioned my moods, wanting to protect me and make sure I wasn't becoming hypomanic.

'Ellie, you're a bit hyper today,' Mum asked me at one point. 'You're talking a lot and you're doing more than usual. Are you okay?'

I shrugged. 'Yeah, I'm fine. I'm just feeling happy, so I want to chat to my friends more. That's all.'

'I need you to make sure you're resting and taking your medication,' Mum replied, looking concerned.

'Nothing's wrong,' I protested. I just wanted to be Ellie, the normal teenager. Couldn't she see that?

'Listen to Mum,' Dad chimed in. 'We're just looking out for you.'

I knew they meant well, but I didn't want to feel different, even though visiting home reminded me that I had changed. I'd had psychosis and panic attacks in my bedroom earlier that year. I had talked to myself in this room; I had sat in my bedroom, believing I was on *Big Brother* and talking to the "cameras". Being here again brought back some difficult memories and gave me flashbacks. Thankfully they passed, and the more I visited home, the more settled I became. Slowly, I began to enjoy being back with my family, although I was still somewhat institutionalised.

My four months in the Priory had been a journey from psychosis to wellness, uncertainty to diagnosis, chaos to calm. I would be under the community CAMHS team after discharge and, armed with their support (along with that of my family), I left with a promise to stick out the medication and therapy. Saying goodbye to the staff upon my discharge was quite poignant, as they'd been there throughout my journey. I left them a gift to say thank you and bade goodbye to some of my friends on the ward.

Things felt a bit scary when my parents drove me home. I had a flicker of hope that I could be well again – but I also wondered when I would be back in hospital. For now, though, I had to learn how to be a teenager living with bipolar disorder.

Now, I needed to look ahead to the future.

CHAPTER 8

ACHIEVING AGAINST THE ODDS

After all that had happened to me, I had a low opinion of myself. I still partly blamed myself for my illness and everything that happened to me in Israel. I was embarrassed that I had wanted to kiss boys I had only just met; it just wasn't in my character.

I didn't know who I was. Who was this teenager with the crazy, uncontrollable brain?

That was the underpinning belief behind my social anxiety. Social anxiety is a form of anxiety or phobia in which you worry that people are going to judge you negatively, and it can lead to panic attacks. My self-esteem was low, and I had a chronic condition that I felt I had no control over at all. Yes, I took medication and yes, I went to therapy. But I didn't have a community around me full of people talking about mental health. Social media was in its infancy. From 2004 to 2006, there was no Facebook, Twitter, or Instagram, and there weren't many blogs or books that I knew of that talked about people like me. There seemed to be nothing I could find for bipolar teenagers either, although there may have been support groups.

I felt like a freak, totally different from everyone around me, who seemed to live carefree lives. They didn't have to take medication or see a psychiatrist. They could drink alcohol like normal teenagers. They didn't have to explain about psychosis, mania or suicidal depression to their friends. They didn't have a social phobia, or if they did, I didn't know about it. I was confused and felt sorry for myself at times, and all of this perpetuated my anxiety about how others perceived me.

After being in hospital, I'd had to go down a year at school to catch up with my A Levels. But at least I was focused again, determined to stay well and apply myself to my recovery. I took my medication and avoided alcohol. I stayed hyper-vigilant and monitored my moods, even if I did overdo it sometimes, stopping myself from having fun at parties or obsessively checking in with myself to see if I was depressed, manic or normal. It was hard to know who Eleanor really was, where the bipolar disorder ended and Eleanor began.

I was still under CAMHS services until I was nineteen, and I had support from a psychiatrist and counsellor. A lot of my close friends had gone into the last year of A Levels, and Charlotte left school to do hers at another college, so I had to make friends in my new year.

One of these friends was Becky. Like me, Becky was new to the school year, having moved for Sixth Form. She was the headmaster's daughter, and we shared a lot of classes. We clicked straight away; we both had a love of literature, stuffed toy animals and 90's chick flicks (*Clueless* and *10 Things I Hate About You* being our favourites). Becky, with her kind face and mischievous brown eyes, helped me feel less alone. She would come and help me get to school when I was anxious, as I lived just down the road. I can't underestimate how important it was to have kind friends around me.

Therapy, friends, and my medical team all helped me settle back into school. I had the sweetest nurse who came into school with me for the first weeks of my A Levels. It was agreed that I would only do a lesson or two a day as I was becoming very tired and my anxiety was sky-high and overwhelming, but over time I slowly built up to more lessons and studying. Mum took time out of work to take me to school and pick me up, feeding me piping-hot tomato soup with rice and buttered toast, making me feel loved and nurtured.

School promoted a caring attitude, and pastoral care was of importance. Most teachers at school were excellent, especially the head of Sixth Form, Dr S. Dr S was one of the most extraordinary teachers I have ever met. He is so well-spoken and well read, with an incredible mind, but it was his warmth and kindness that stood out. In school he dressed immaculately in suits and polished shoes, but outside he was more of a rebel; he had piercings and rode a motorcycle. We absolutely loved it when we found out.

Dr S was so supportive; he would regularly call me into his office for a chat to see how I was doing. He knew about my mental illness and that I had spent time in hospital, and he and his team were so kind to me. Without his advice and the help of my other teachers, I would have found it much harder to apply for university.

Despite what had happened with my drama GCSE, I still had the acting bug. My mental health was more stable and my moods were on an even keel. I kept appointments with my psychiatrist and took my medicine. I felt less vulnerable, less overly emotional and more confident in my ability to act again. I had been in five plays over my five years at school, so I decided to audition again.

I cherished my role as Lady Bracknell in *The Importance of Being Earnest* by Oscar Wilde. Lady Bracknell is a formidable lady of the aristocracy and is the main character's grandmother. She's a hilarious character, the true matriarch of the piece. She was completely different to me. With her, I was stepping into an unusual world, escaping into her story, perfecting her mannerisms. With her, I didn't have to focus on my own mental health struggles.

I was known at school for being the one who loved acting – if my story was in an American movie, I would be part of the drama clique, the geek trying her best to impress the drama teachers at every audition. You could give me a script and I'd be happy.

At lunch time, I could often be found running around in costume advertising the school productions with the rest of the cast. One time I wore a lilac and pink Victorian hat that I would wear when playing Lady Bracknell. Playing such a well-loved and famous hero of literature filled me with pride.

I thrived on the art of performing and crafting a character. In many ways, the escapism helped me when my own life was in turmoil. And so, when it came to choosing my degree, there was only one choice.

Going to uni was a huge deal for me. I had applied to London universities – UCL, Kings, Queen Mary and Goldsmiths, University of London – to study English literature. The course at Goldsmiths was joint with drama and this drew me to it, but my first choice was to study English at UCL.

While getting rejected from both UCL and Kings was upsetting – they were such good universities – it was a real blessing in disguise. I was offered places at Queen Mary to do English and the joint Drama and English Literature degree at Goldsmiths. I was overjoyed to have the option to study drama alongside another subject. I would go on to study acting theory, undertake practical acting (much like the work of Stanislavski and Brecht), read plays, and study world theatre, including Spanish and African. I'd also read English literature.

Not only that, but past alumni included Mary Quant (creator of the mini skirt), Julian Clary, and Damien Hirst. Even Princess Beatrice attended, the year after me. If we had been in the same year, the Queen would have been at my graduation! I was sad to have missed her – I'm a fan of the monarchy and all the charity work they do, especially for mental illness. The princess tended to keep a low profile at university, but I once saw her by the drama theatre with her security guard, and that excited me. I was proud to be attending an institution that had so many successful, creative people and alumni, and I hoped that I would follow in their (very big) footsteps.

I knew it in my gut: Goldsmiths was right place for me, and going to the open day confirmed that. As Mum and I walked up to the impressive Richard Hoggart building and were taken on guided tours around the campus and library – ending with a lecture in the hall on the English course, something clicked. I can't put my finger on whether it was the relaxed, arts-school creative atmosphere or the unique heritage, but I wanted to study there. Impressed by its emphasis on individuality, creative arts and expressing oneself, I worked hard to make sure I got a place.

The doctors at the Priory had said that I may not ever be able to go to university because bipolar is a chronic condition, with my type (bipolar 1) being the most serious, so I was just ecstatic that I got such good grades in my A Levels and that my perseverance had paid off. I was filled with excitement, feeling more like a normal teenager. I couldn't wait to start my course.

But I was also battling the anxiety.

There is a misconception that social anxiety means you are cripplingly shy and can't make friends, but this isn't true for everyone. Sometimes it's just hard for people to show their friendliness due to the anxiety – and sometimes, like me, you can have friends but also feel anxious at the same time.

This was a big step for me, as Goldsmiths is based in New Cross, South London, and I lived at home in Hertfordshire. The journey was about an hour and a half by car.

I was almost nineteen, and I'd had such a turbulent few years. Thankfully my mum and dad were still there to look out for me; Mum even made sure we did a practice run of my journey to Goldsmiths on the Tube. I was so grateful to have her. Mum was completely selfless and she would do anything to make sure I felt confident and settled, even as a nineteen-year-old woman. In truth, I still felt like a scared child in many ways because of my social anxiety and panic attacks, but I craved independence. I wanted to learn how to cook properly, to buy my own shopping, to live away from home. I wanted to see what else was out there, to prove I could do it on my own and be happy. I hadn't done a gap year like a lot of people at my school; instead, I'd spent my time in a psychiatric hospital and recovering at home. For these reasons, living at university and making new friends was important to me. I would still be in London, but I would be able to create my own life.

And so finally, in 2007, I walked up to the beautiful, red-brick Richard Hoggart Building on the Goldsmiths Campus. I was awestruck, although registering was a bit nerve-wracking. There were so many people, and I had to go from building to building, winding my way through the black tiled-floor corridors, in order to register at both the English and drama departments.

I was in the queue to register, nervously clutching my registration details, when I saw a girl dressed in black-and-white skeleton leggings, a leather jacket and long boots. To top it off, she was also wearing a plastic skull necklace. She had sleek, strawberry-blonde hair and a cheeky smile, and she was speaking to someone else in the queue about the fact that she was starting English and drama. I turned to her shyly and said, 'I'm also doing English and drama. What's your name? I'm Eleanor – I created the freshers' group on Facebook.'

The girl turned to me with a grin on her face. 'Wow, nice to meet you. I think we've spoken online already! I'm George. Excuse me for sitting on the radiator; I'm cold and I've just had a cup of coffee to keep warm, but it's making me jittery!'

George's personality was infectious, and I instantly warmed to her. She was simply hilarious, and we became fast friends. Like me, George travelled to uni from home and wasn't living in halls, so in the first term we travelled together on the Tube a lot. We had a shared joke about the place "Rotherhithe" being pronounced "Ro'hithe" in a pirate voice, complete with hand actions (you had to be there, clearly).

I also met other people on our course who were fab, including Hayleigh, a lovely girl from the Welsh Valleys; Hannah from Stroud, who was a bundle of fun; and Sophie, who was a kindly, mature student. We all sat together in English lectures, which were held in a massive hall with hundreds of people. The induction lecture was daunting – we were asked to read a huge selection of books including one classic book a week. (I must confess that I didn't read every book set ...)

It was fun getting to know plenty of people across the two departments; there were hundreds of students on the English course and only forty on the drama course. There were about thirty of us doing the joint degree and we all stuck together. I had to miss some early lectures due to the Jewish festivals, as our high holy days begin to take place around that time, but I managed to catch up quickly.

But before we could start our course properly, we had freshers' week. Given that I have social anxiety, it might come as a surprise that I'd gone out of my way to make friends online before university, but I have always been very friendly and that gave me confidence. I met Jenni and Nicola, two fellow students that I'd met through the Facebook group for students starting in 2007. Nicola was also from Bushey (though our paths had never crossed) and she was studying English and drama too.

We all decided to dress up as the Spice Girls, as it was a 90s themed night in the student union bar. I was dressed as Scary Spice, wearing leopard-print leggings, as the other girls had taken Baby and Ginger. I don't know what we were thinking – we even got up on stage to sing a karaoke version of 'Wannabe'! We'd not had any alcohol, so it wasn't even like we were drunk. The older students were smiling and laughing at us, giving us bemused looks, clearly thinking we freshers were rather amusing as the only ones in fancy dress – but that was why we'd decided to do it.

I felt I needed to embrace this new opportunity with wild abandon, with new friends in a new atmosphere. These people didn't know I had been in hospital as a teenager, so I could create a somewhat new identity at the beginning. Everyone was so friendly, and I felt like I was really fitting in.

New Cross is quite an eclectic area, especially the high street. I used to love walking past the shops – one of the best being a fashion shop run by students – and cosy pubs. Our favourite haunt was The Hobgoblin by our halls, which had the loveliest garden, and we'd also sit and have a few drinks in The Amersham Arms, a very quirky place with interesting clocks and artefacts on the walls. Behind The Hobgoblin and our halls was the famous Goldsmiths art building, an extremely beautiful addition to the London skyline. Not only does it spell out "GOLDSMITHS" in capital letters, but there is a sculpture on top shaped like a reel of film tape. It's stunning.

The university is specialist in arts subjects and is very much a liberal arts school. It was commonplace at the time (and I imagine now too) to see people with multi-coloured or bright hair (anything went – bright blue, red, green) or wearing vintage dresses and red lipstick to lectures. Some of my fellow drama students loved expressing themselves in this way; piercings and artistic tattoos were also commonplace. Skinny jeans were very popular for both men and women. One time, I was served in the university shop by a man wearing goggles on his head!

I loved this self-expression. It was very different to what I'd known at school. Immanuel College is a traditional Orthodox Jewish school, and during my time there, it had been all about being properly groomed and fitting in. A lot of people wore designer labels or had expensive bags and shoes, and everyone straightened their hair or tamed their curls so that it was shiny and sleek. Most girls wore make-up daily. In Sixth Form, we had to dress smartly; boys wore suits and girls had to wear skirts or dresses, in keeping with Orthodox Judaism. No one really had bright hair or any piercings or tattoos on show. "Coming out" at school rarely happened, largely due to the time period (early 2000s) and the fact that we are a small, religious community. In fact, the majority of my LGBT friends came out after school. LGBT issues were discussed a bit at school, but many people felt they could not be openly gay there (though I'm sure the teachers would have been supportive). I'm sure things have changed now.

School didn't stifle me, but because I had to become hyper-vigilant with my illness and moods, I didn't have a chance to reinvent or build on my identity. This is why Goldsmiths felt like the right place for me: it was different. It was freeing. Goldsmiths gave me a chance to find out who Eleanor really was. I have never been a rebel and I have always tried to look after myself for my mental health, so Goldsmiths allowed me to indulge in that bit of rebellion I'd been missing. It was okay to be straight, bi, or gay, to have pink or green hair, to have lots of tattoos or piercings. It was okay to wear vintage fashion and to study music or drama.

In the first term, I socialised a lot with new friends in their flat in Loring Hall, one of the main halls of residence by the campus. We'd go to the student union together for bar nights, and I'd sit with them in lectures (writing notes to each other when we got bored). We'd watch trashy TV in our spare time (often accompanied by pizza, pesto pasta or hot chocolate – the staple student diet). So, now that I was having so much fun with my friends, I decided that I wanted to live at university too, as I was missing out on the experience. So I applied to Loring Hall and was told that I could move in in the January. I was thrilled! This would be my first time living away from home independently and I couldn't wait.

This wasn't the entire story, though. This was a big step, and I was a bit concerned – I still had anxiety issues, and I was still learning how to deal with the increased level of panic. My panic attacks would last for about fifteen minutes, after which I would often fall asleep to escape what was happening. Sometimes I would hyperventilate, run away or hide in my bedroom if I was too scared to leave the house. Tears would roll down my cheeks and I'd go hot and clammy as the adrenaline soared through my veins. My social anxiety meant that some days I didn't want to be around people.

On the other hand, having an illness like bipolar disorder can make you feel dependent on others to help you through, so it was great for me to have that space and independence to deal with everything I had been through.

My new flatmates were an eclectic bunch and I loved sharing a flat with them all. One was a music student and aspiring musician; two others were on my English course and loved all things quirky, vintage and artistic; one was from Russia studying media and taught me a lot about Russian culture (although she loved *EastEnders*); another was studying politics and was really down-to-earth. We'd chat about our lives or the latest music at two o'clock in the morning when we couldn't sleep, and we'd cook together while having our daily catchups. When I was bored, I decorated our kitchen noticeboard with pictures of celebrities we loved – including Justin Timberlake, of course. One time, one of my male flatmates declared a water-bomb war on the flat above. I hid in my room while it was happening, but when I heard the commotion outside, I came out just in time to see that the flat above had somehow got into our kitchen and were throwing sour milk around. The smell the next day made me feel so sick! We all insisted that our flatmate clear it up – and he did, to his credit. Oh, uni life ...

I enjoyed most of my lectures. For our acting classes, we had to wear a black top and tracksuit bottoms or leggings. Staff insisted upon us wearing black so that we could start performing from a neutral, authentic place. It was great to have classes in the Goldsmiths theatre with tutors who were experts in their field. Some were actors and acting coaches in their own right. In our first year we had to create modern and experimental theatre pieces that included the techniques we were learning, such as mime, for example. In one, I and six other people played evil trees, to the amusement of my family. What an unusual performance! I was in my element.

I had the best time in first year. I knew that there were Jewish students at Goldsmiths, but compared to other London universities, they were far less actively involved in Jewish life on campus. It was important to me that I joined the Jewish Society (or "J-Soc") because I wanted to make Jewish friends at university, share cultural and religious events, and help other Jewish people, some of whom were far from home. In one of my first weeks, I contacted the society's head, Rivka, and as I was walking down the tiled corridors towards the Loafers Café, I saw a few men with kippot (Jewish head coverings). There were a few girls with them too.

I nervously approached and asked them if they were part of J-Soc.

'Yes!' one of them replied eagerly. 'Who are you?'

'Hi, my name's Eleanor,' I said, introducing myself, and we proceeded to play a game of "Jewish geography". This meant that we all found out each other's last names, which schools we had gone to, and if we knew anyone in common. Usually people do, and this makes things much easier, since being Jewish is a bit like having an extended family. It turned out that Rivka had gone to school with people I knew. She introduced me to Daniel, her lovely co-chair; Yossi, who was a mature student studying psychology; Eleanor, who had long dark hair and a bright smile; and Leonie, who was a German student studying drama. We all instantly connected.

We discussed life on campus and how I could get involved with J-Soc. I soon realised that, since Goldsmiths students were liberal and sometimes held views on the far left about Israel and politics, it was difficult to be Jewish on campus. There was no overt anti-Semitism as such, but the Palestine Solidarity Campaign was quite rife on campus, calling for boycotts of Israeli people, goods and products, and regularly holding protests. When I became involved with J-Soc in my first term, Yossi and I tried to combat the misconceptions we heard and form a dialogue with people on campus. We expressed our feelings about people's comparisons between the Holocaust and Israel's treatment of Palestinians. Most of us had lost relatives in the Holocaust and so it was an emotive topic. It wasn't easy, but it was a part of J-Soc life.

In my second year, I became assistant head of J-Soc, with Yossi as head. We put on fun events, such "Lunch and Learn" with Rabbi Dovid Cohen and Rabbi Gavin Broder (the London Chaplain), restaurant nights out to kosher places in Golders Green, Chanukah parties, and regular get-togethers. On Friday nights, we'd meet up for dinner at Hillel House in Euston with the other London J-Socs. We also promoted places and events for our members to spend the Jewish festivals if they didn't have family around. I adored being involved with J-Soc, despite the difficulties on our campus surrounding Israel.

My friends had graduated by my third year, but new people from all across the world joined our J-Soc. I became head, which was exciting, and I was involved in organising events for London J-Socs, such as the famous "Booze for Jews" bar night. On average, we must have had about twenty or thirty people attending our campus events. This sounds small, but we were a small society! I thrived on promoting our society at the Freshers' Fair, communicating on social media and email with our members and creating events for them. It was a special time. I met people from all over the world, spending time with friends old and new, and I felt so involved in Jewish life!

There was still a lot going on in my life, but university was an important distraction. It helped keep my mind off my broken heart.

CHAPTER 9

EMBRACING MY JEWISH IDENTITY

The summer before uni, Joe and I had met up again. We'd always had a strong connection and we'd stayed in touch, often through long phone calls. And so we started dating again, becoming inseparable throughout that summer. It feels odd to me that I was in love at nineteen years old, but I was.

We did normal teenage things, visiting the cinema and going out for late-night drives. We went up to London a few times and even went on a night-time boat cruise on the Thames. I loved spending time with him, and we had happy times together, but it was clear that we didn't work well in a romantic relationship. We would argue about our values, about things we wanted. I wasn't ready to settle down yet – I was only nineteen and I was still studying! – but Joe was working and wanted to get married. He also had his own struggles in life, and while I tried, I just couldn't help him. Still, it devastated me when we broke up.

I cried my eyes out. I missed him so much. *Why has he abandoned me?* I'd think, angry and hurt at the situation. The only way I got through it was having friends listen to me as I cried, supplying me with chocolate and hugs.

Soon after we broke up, Joe got engaged to someone else. I was shocked. How had this happened? He'd been *my* boyfriend just a few months earlier, and he'd only been dating his new girlfriend for a short time. He was my first love, and I did want to marry him at some point, just not at that moment! I'd imagined being his wife many times, picturing a future and projecting all my hopes onto him. We had spoken about building a home and a family; I just didn't want that until I'd graduated. He'd even met my parents and told them of his intention to marry me one day.

The rug was pulled out from underneath me when I saw his wedding photos on Facebook a few months later. It hurt – a lot. I tried to be happy for him and his new wife, but all I felt was confusion, misunderstanding, and a whole lot of pain in both my head and my heart. Was all that I'd felt, and all that he'd said to me, a lie? We'd been through a lot together. How could I carry on when the love of my life had left? It was obvious that he wanted to build a family and he wasn't coming back. I was truly, intensely, overwhelmingly heartbroken. It almost felt like I was in physical pain, as though I'd been kicked in my stomach. My heart was in pieces and I felt broken, emotionally exhausted. It took me months to recover.

With hindsight, I can see that although I loved Joe dearly, he was much better suited to being my friend rather than a partner. Our feelings had come at the wrong time in our lives, when we both were so young and couldn't deal with it. Timing is everything. I know he feels the same as me.

My family picked me up when I was feeling low, and they made sure that I was sleeping, eating and looking after myself. And despite the agony, I believed strongly that whatever pain I was going through, it would get better. I felt lost at times, but working hard at university helped save me too. Creating theatre, reading plays and books, studying for my exams and going out with my friends got me through it. It helped that I was living away from people who knew me at home.

It was a combination of Joe leaving and me feeling so desolate that led me to up my observance level with Judaism. I had grown up in a traditional, Orthodox family, but as I was exploring my religion more, I realised I wanted to keep kosher fully and keep the Sabbath fully along with other tenets of my religion. I decided to dress more modestly and give up my beloved jeans (there is an Orthodox Jewish rule that women should wear skirts and dresses to be modest, and cover their elbows, collar bone and knee).

I wanted to embrace Judaism and God more because I had been through so much in my short life that it helped me make sense of who I was, my identity and what I needed spiritually and emotionally. I found comfort in religion, and I still do when I pray. I knew there was a greater plan for me and knowing that God was there helped in my healing process. I began to pray more and learn more Jewishly, reading the Tenach (Bible) and Jewish self-development and dating books.

I needed to be on antidepressants and I was seeing a new psychiatrist again. My social anxiety was closely linked to my self-esteem issues, and I needed to address that. My anxiety had become intense. I felt rejected – I *had* been rejected – and I felt like I wasn't worthy or good enough.

Social occasions began to spark panic attacks. One night, I received a text from a friend. 'Ellie, we're going out to a bar tomorrow night. Come with us!'

I looked blankly at the screen as my heart quickened. I didn't want to go. I didn't want to put on make-up, smile and fake being happy. I didn't want people looking at me or talking to me. I just wanted to hide.

'Sorry, I'm not feeling well, so I can't come. But I'll see you soon.'

The relief flooded through me. No one would judge me negatively for this. I'd be safe indoors and, since this was still a preoccupation of mine after my manic episode, I was relieved that I wouldn't get unwanted male attention.

I went through this level of panic every time anyone asked me to a social occasion. Occasionally, if a friend probed or wouldn't leave me alone, my panic would worsen. Fight-or-flight mode would kick in and I'd hide away in my bedroom – my place of safety. I'd tuck myself under my blanket and sleep to block out the anxiety. I was still barely older than a teenager and still learning to cope with my bipolar diagnosis too, which wasn't easy. I desperately needed extra support.

Cognitive behavioural therapy had helped my dad get better, so I decided that I needed to go to counselling too in order to help my social phobia and the trauma of being unwell, being hospitalised, and being heartbroken by all that had gone on with Joe.

My therapist, Linda, was a sweet, Northern, Jewish lady who lived near me. She understood my cultural background, which was important because I needed a therapist who had a good knowledge of my religion and the stigmas in the Jewish world at that time. My community didn't fully understand what I was going through because it wasn't talked about openly, and I didn't know any other teenagers like me in the Jewish world. (Of course, there will have been others, but I didn't know that then.) Linda practised CBT, talking therapy and EMDR (Eye Movement Desensitisation and Processing), which is meant to help process trauma through the process of tapping on certain points on the body and using eye movements.

I spent a couple of months with her, talking about everything that had gone on, but also working on the social anxiety by challenging my thoughts in thought records. Those thoughts were often worries that my peers were scrutinising me and going to reject me. I had been cancelling a lot of arrangements with my friends as I felt an overwhelming fear that I wasn't good enough. Some of them understood and were amazingly supportive; they would come to my house anyway and show me love and kindness. Sometimes, though, my friends didn't understand it, especially if I had to cancel going to an important event like a birthday or engagement. People don't see why you can't always push through with anxiety, because it's not tangible.

To help me process the trauma of being unwell, my therapist used some EMDR techniques with me, which involved my focusing on a difficult memory while she helped me to process it using rapid eye movements. Much like in REM sleep, where the sleeper's eyes move rapidly, this helps clear the subconscious mind of the traumatic experience and to process it through rapid processing in the brain. EMDR activates both hemispheres of the brain at the same time, which is meant to help process a trauma over time. It is often used in the treatment of post-traumatic stress disorder, although I have never been diagnosed with it.

It was helpful to talk about what had gone on and to attempt the CBT techniques. There are different kinds, but in general, CBT is an action-based therapy that is meant to help change negative thought processes and behaviour. Unfortunately, it didn't seem to help my social phobia. I couldn't implement the positive thoughts because I would get overwhelmed with panic attacks. My anxiety became so heightened that I'd just freeze – I couldn't stop it. I did find recording my thoughts to be useful sometimes, though. I would challenge my beliefs on paper and try to replace them with positive thoughts.

The therapy did help my depression. It was good to be heard and to have that weekly session to talk about everything, and my therapist was very patient. I also continued to practise self-care to stay well. I loved to read, pray, and write in my journal. I wrote a lot of poetry, which helped me make sense of my emotions and broken heart. I saw my close friends when I could, and we'd have girly evenings watching movies. I went to therapy and took my medicine as prescribed. I socialised with my friends in halls when I felt able to. University really helped take my mind off things and I slowly began to be feel less anxious, although I still worried about having sudden panic attacks. In one such attack, a friend popped in to see me without telling me, which triggered irrational panic. My anxiety was so high that I stood at the door, barricading it, making sure that my friend wouldn't see me. This type of panic was debilitating, but slowly it improved.

Yes, I'd been through so much. I had lost the man I was in love with. I'd had to deal with rejection. I'd had to get my head around him getting married very soon after our relationship had ended. But this whole experience taught me that sometimes in life, people either make choices, or God intervenes. It has taught me that, while going through a breakup and serious mental illness was a nightmare at times, I could survive the pain and heartbreak.

I know now that Joe leaving my life had a purpose, even if I couldn't see it then. I prayed to God to help me get through it.

In time, my family, my faith, and my friends would bring me to the light.

CHAPTER 10

BUILDING CONFIDENCE THROUGH
THE WONDER OF TRAVEL

I was still missing Joe dearly, but I was beginning to recover again – so much so that I felt strong enough to go with my school friends Anna, Katie and Hannah on a trip to India during the university summer break in 2008. This was a milestone for me; it represented freedom, exploration and wonder. I was so excited, and it proved to be incredibly healing.

The trip was an absolute whirlwind. It boosted my health and made me feel empowered. We went all over the country, trying to see as much as we could in just three weeks, and although we planned our route while in England, we couldn't have understood the beauty and madness that was India until we arrived.

India has a vastly different culture to the UK. We went in June, during the monsoon season, which meant that we experienced the wet heat mixed with the buzzing of mosquitoes, the delicious smells of spices cooking, brightly coloured clothing and friendly people. Sadly, we also saw a lot of poverty; there were beggars hungry for food and in need of money, disabled people on the streets without access to wheelchairs, and workers sleeping on the floor outside our hotel rooms. It was harrowing to witness; I felt quite guilty for being a tourist when there was so much poverty. Sometimes I gave my food away to children or women with babies who asked us, but we had to be careful not to give to everyone or we would get swamped – we learnt this the hard way at a market one day.

Despite our sadness about the poverty, I had a brilliant time with my friends. Anna is my second cousin and we have all known each other since we were eleven years old, so we were a tight-knit group who looked out for each other. They knew that I would have to take my bipolar medication regularly and stay well rested. Still quite paranoid about becoming manic, I made sure to sleep a lot (despite the heat and mosquitoes) and drink lots of bottled water to avoid dehydration. I avoided alcohol and checked in a lot with my friends to see if my moods seemed normal. I was completely fine, but I was vigilant with myself; I was concerned that what happened in Israel could happen again. I did not want to become hyper-sexual or out of control with mania again, but as the days passed, I learnt to relax and realise I could enjoy myself without something bad happening.

In Delhi, we saw beautiful ancient palaces and rode elephants. We saw forts, tea shops, mosques and temples. We visited the famous Taj Mahal at Agra and went on a tiger safari at Ranthambore National Park (it took seven hours to get there and we didn't get to see any tigers, though we saw elephants and other animals). We stayed in Pushkar, a mountain town with lots of monkeys and a tranquil lake, which is holy for Hindus. After Pushkar, we went into Rajasthan State – which is filled with palaces and beautiful historical buildings – to visit Jaipur, the city of pink stone, where we visited carpet shops and palaces, swam in our hotel pool and learnt about its history. We saw the Hawa Mahal, the vast, pink "Palace of the Winds", with its curved arches and lattice design. We stayed in a plush hotel, complete with Indian wall hangings, fabric and marble, a vast contrast to the poverty we saw on the streets.

From Jaipur we flew to Mumbai where, on my twentieth birthday, as we were celebrating in a café and eating chocolate birthday cake, we were asked to be extras in a real Bollywood movie with movie star Shahid Kapoor. It's an experience I will never forget.

A well-groomed man with a flashy silver watch came over to our table as we were eating. 'Excuse me, girls,' he said. 'I'm Imran, and I work in the Bollywood film industry. We are shooting a film just outside Mumbai tomorrow, and need Western extras to join us in the background on set. There are already a few from England and Italy on board. Would you like to join us? If so, meet us on the main street tomorrow at two o'clock in the afternoon.' He then handed me his business card.

My friends looked at me bemused. 'We'll need to talk about it, but I think we would love to,' I said, hesitantly. 'But how do we know you're really in Bollywood? And is it a paid opportunity?'

Imran smiled and pointed to a web address on his business card. 'Look me up, and you'll see I am a real agent,' he replied. 'You will get paid in rupees. Hope to see you all tomorrow.'

Most of us were sceptical. Were we really being asked to be in Bollywood – and on my birthday? As it turned out, yes. It was a real opportunity, and there was a famous Bollywood star featuring in the movie, so we all bundled into a van and drove to the outskirts of Mumbai. We worked a twelve-hour day for the equivalent of twenty pence – thankfully we knew this, and we didn't mind the cost as it was a special experience). Due to filming, we didn't get on set until midnight, so we stayed in the holding tent, chatting to the other extras and eating curry.

The film was set in Australia and we were extras in the nightclub set, dancing in the background and chatting to the Indian actors as the camera passed. I was on cloud nine. Here I was, studying drama at university and spending time on a Bollywood film set – even if it was in a field on the outskirts of Mumbai! My friends were excited too – it was a real "once-in-a-lifetime" experience. We finished the shoot at two o'clock in the morning and went back to our hotel to sleep.

The next morning, I woke up and looked at the clock. It was 6 am.

I quickly came to a jolt. We were due to fly to Kerala at 7.30 am! Everyone was still curled up in their duvets, having succumbed to the lull of sleep after our night of glitter and fun. I gently shook the girls awake. 'Wake up! We've overslept!' I told them urgently. 'It's already six o'clock! We're going to miss our flight!'

They looked at me with tired, bemused expressions before it dawned on them – we were late, and over an hour away from the airport!

Hurriedly we threw our belongings into bags, pulling on clothes and checking out as fast as we could. We managed to hail a taxi to take us to the airport, and by the time we got there, the staff had given away our economy seats. It worked out great, though, because by the time we'd explained what had happened, we'd been upgraded to business class! We laughed so hard at the irony of the day – our lateness had been rewarded with an upgrade to footrests and luxury seats!

And so we flew to southern India ...

Kerala, India's most southern state – and our last stop – was a picturesque, tropical landscape with coconut trees. It is home to pineapple plants, rice paddy fields, and the biggest freshwater lake in the country. We stayed in a little homestay with a wonderful family who cooked curries for us. While there we toured the lakes – known as "the backwaters" – each day, stopping at the sides to explore the villages and meet the people who lived along the river. We went to the beach, saw some elephants and had henna patterns swirled over our palms and feet. It was a gorgeous, relaxed place. The culture was rich and vibrant, and we were given amazing hospitality from local people. We felt safe there.

This trip changed my life and boosted my confidence. It had only been four years since I had been in hospital, yet here I was, exercising that independence that university had given me. India helped me further explore my identity and experience new and varied things under the guidance and support of my friends. Here, I didn't have to worry about the grind of everyday life. Here, I could be young and happy and free.

For the third year of university in 2009 and 2010, I moved from halls to live in North London with Anna and her family, as they lived nearer to the university. This was a wonderful time in my life during which we hosted friends and family frequently. I wasn't living at home in Hertfordshire, but I still went home to spend time with my mum and dad, and Chantal was living on the same road as me, so I got to see her a lot too.

After I had finished my final university exams, I went on another trip with Anna, Katie and Hannah – this time to Tamale, Ghana. It was a volunteering trip, and it changed my perspective for the better.

I had wanted to go and visit Africa for a while, ever since I'd read a special book called *Born on the Continent: Ubuntu* by my friend, Getrude Matshe. Getrude is an entrepreneur, author and international speaker, who set up the Africa Alive Education Foundation to help her child relatives and friends who were orphaned due to the AIDS epidemic in Zimbabwe. My friends and I saw that a Jewish social action charity named Tzedek were running a seven-week trip to volunteer in communities in Northern Ghana, so we jumped at the chance. We'd had an amazing experience in India, but now we wanted to make a difference (however small) and learn more about life beyond the confines of middle-class North West London.

We all had our interviews at the Tzedek headquarters, where they assessed our interests for placements and whether we would be right for the trip. We also met the four others who would be going to Ghana with us. I love working with children and was happy to work with other women, so I was overjoyed to be assigned GIGDEV (Girls Growth and Development) as my placement.

GIGDEV is an NGO (non-governmental organisation) set up to help vulnerable women known as "Kayaye Girls". These women come from poor backgrounds and are in search of work. When they get to Accra, the capital, they are often abused or raped and live in terrible conditions. Some fall pregnant at a young age. GIGDEV was set up to help those girls who come back to the north – some are only fifteen or sixteen years old. It teaches them a trade (either hairdressing or dressmaking) so that they can start their own business and earn money. Many of the women are illiterate, so they have an hour each day of learning to read English and basic maths skills. Their children are cared for in the on-site nursery.

Volunteering with the charity had a profound impact on me. I adored helping the staff and playing with the children, and every morning I would come in to teach my class for an hour. I would witness them all go from smiling, laughing and joking to super serious and eager to learn. I wasn't a qualified teacher, but I was able to teach them basic English words and arithmetic.

Here is an extract from my Ghana diary:

We arrived here in Tamale three weeks ago, and so much has happened since we have been here.

The other seven volunteers and I are staying in a house in the little village of Fuo, next to SSNIT, a suburb of Tamale. It is quite far from the majority of our placements – which are past the centre of town – and we have to get two taxis to get to work every day. The taxis often leave much to be desired, but we all cram into them every day. To get to the taxis we walk past mud huts and goats, and the villagers call out to us. Sometimes they shout, 'Siliminga!' (white person) or 'Desba!' (good morning!) with smiles and waves. The culture here is to greet everyone who approaches you and so walking through the village gives you a very warm feeling. Every morning we see the old man at the side of the road tending to his crops, the young school boy riding his bicycle on his way to school, a group of girls giggling, and the woman at the side of the road selling egg bread or cooked maize, all while dodging the dust, goat poo, motorbikes and potential muddy puddles!

Tamale is a welcoming and friendly place. There have been many challenges, including a lack of cooking gas in the first week, trying to build a fire when it randomly pours with torrential rain, and the guilty feeling of being in a Westernised house (albeit built by a Ghanaian) while some of those around us live in mud with straw and animals roaming free. It didn't feel right at first but what was pointed out was that we couldn't have successfully got through our experience without certain facilities. I feel privileged to be living in this village and seeing another way of life, even though it can feel uncomfortable at times. A volunteer in a previous year mentioned that one feels like a celebrity as a white person here, and it's true. Children in particular get very excited when they see you, and you are highly visible, however adapted you feel to the culture around you.

We began our placements after touring central Tamale and acquainting ourselves with the area and a couple of NGOs. I am working at GIGDEV, which takes impoverished girls, some who have had to drop out of school because of teen pregnancy, some who went to the south of the country looking for work but ended up doing menial tasks, and others who come from difficult backgrounds. GIGDEV is a sustainable development organisation promoting self-help, education and rights for women and children. It focuses on the marginalised in society, providing them with vocational skills such as dressmaking and hairdressing, so they can start their own businesses and get out of poverty. The hope for the Kayaye Girls is that they will stay in the northern region and give back to their local communities rather than go off for a fruitless search for work down south in Accra.

I am working at GIGDEV as a literacy, numeracy and IT teacher for women aged between fifteen and twenty-five. I also worked in the nursery – "Kiddicare" – for three weeks until it closed for the summer, assisting the teachers and looking after the children. This was an eye-opening experience because I came into contact with the first use of the cane here. It shocked me that children so young were being caned, but this is the disciplinary system here. I couldn't intervene, but the teacher caning felt that they had to justify it to me continuously, as they know the cane is now banned in England.

The teachers were lovely women and we shared some fun moments. We sang African songs while the three-year-olds came up to dance one by one, swaying from side to side. We taught the children maths (which is more difficult than it sounds with poor resources) and played with the children in the playground, sorting out their fights and scrapes! My friend Rachel and I became "hello girls" because the kids would jump on us and shout, 'Hello, hello, hello!' to us as we entered the class.

I am finding teaching the women so rewarding – though I wish I had more time to teach them than just one hour a day! I hope they're benefiting, even on a small level. It's special to be able to teach women around my age and build relationships with people from a different culture. I will treasure it for the rest of my life. It's fascinating to see their reactions to what I teach them, whether that be a song (as it was today), or reading, or English verbs, or fractions ...

I have also been taking part in an after-school club at Morning Star, a school for orphans and poorer children in the community. This has been an amazing experience – and also a wake-up call. Morning Star is made up of little shacks with blackboards, small wooden desks and no electric lighting. There are incredibly basic resources here, but the after-school club has been wonderful. We run it for an hour and a half every afternoon on a week day, and the children can choose between sport, drama, art, reading, maths, or whatever we decide to run on the day. I have been largely involved with playing drama games with the children, and they are currently working on two plays: Teen Pregnancy (this play warns about the dangers of teen pregnancy; it's a big big problem amongst the poor in the north, and it was suggested as a topic by the children themselves) and The Wicked Stepmother, a more traditional fairy story with African elements. It has been great building relationship with the children. It makes me happy to see them get so excited when we teach them a new game or when I see how much a child loves to act. We have found genuine acting talent!

Like I said, there have been wake-up calls, such as when the children ask me for water because they don't have any at home and they become dehydrated (temperatures get up to 40 degrees here). Or child became so hungry they started eating a plant leaf. I felt so torn. On the one hand, you want to give the children some food, but *on the other, you know that if you do, the expectation will always be there to give them more, and then the forty or so other children will want food too. It's a difficult conundrum, one that some of us face on a daily basis.*

Ghana is eye-opening, enriching, challenging, difficult and amazing all at once. There is so much to write about – the boys playing football in the village, going to an African wedding, our excursion to a Tamale nightclub for our friends' birthdays … and the list goes on …

Ghana helped change me as a person. I learnt that I didn't need as many Western luxuries, and that education, healthcare, provisions and infrastructure are so important to a country, especially one like Ghana. The poverty was stark, and I resolved to make a difference – even if only in a small way – when I came home. While there, I donated books and pens to GIGDEV for its pupils and also gave them my mosquito net in the hope it would help in the battle against the malaria that is prevalent there. Many of the volunteers did this; we wanted to do all we could to help our new friends.

For my thirtieth birthday, some eight years later, I resolved to help GIGDEV after I received an email, asking if I could help fund a shop that would sustain the NGO. It was a project close to my heart, and incredibly, my friends donated £500, which went far after the currency conversion from pounds to Ghanaian cedis. The money was enough to repaint and rewire the shop and stock it with water bottles, clothing and jewellery to sell. It is our hope that the money made from this will be channelled back into the NGO to help more incredible women get a job and education at GIGDEV.

Travelling with friends helped me to tap into my own power and changed my outlook on life. It gave me strength and freedom, teaching me that my life was not only about bipolar disorder. I *could* go abroad without getting sick like I had when I was sixteen.

I'd confirmed it for myself: my life *could* be rich with positive experiences.

CHAPTER 11

DEALING WITH DIVORCE

It was September 2010, and I was staring up again at the red-brick Richard Hoggart Building on the Goldsmiths Campus. I'd recently returned from Ghana and was due to embark on life as a new graduate. Today was my graduation day, a momentous occasion for me.

I had found out from a course mate that I had achieved a 2:1 degree in Drama and English, and I was so thrilled. I had worked hard on all my exams, writing my dissertation 'The Theatre of the Holocaust and Anti-Semitism on Stage'. It was a very moving and powerful – though harrowing – subject to research, and I was proud of what I had put together (despite needing endless cups of tea and chocolate!). The project reaffirmed the journey my family and so many others had been on, under the shadow of the Holocaust.

Frustratingly, my original graduation date had clashed with our Jewish High Holy Days (Rosh Hashana). This meant that I couldn't attend with my course mates as I was with family in synagogue, so I ended up graduating with the music graduates. Mum, Dad and Chantal came with me on the Tube all the way to New Cross to see me put on my black cap and gown (it was very Harry Potter – thankfully I didn't trip in my heels or drop my hat), walk across the stage in front of other students and their families, and shake hands with the chancellor. It meant a lot to have them with me on my important day. Mum still likes to say that the graduation was "so Goldsmiths" – she just loved that there were hippy creative parents there with rainbow-coloured hair, just like their kids.

It was nice to relax in the marquee afterwards with a drink in hand, toasting our three years. Sadly, though, this is a bit marred by the fact that it was one of the last happy times that I remember of my parents still being together.

I was sad to be leaving Goldsmiths, but I felt ready to enter the big wide world of work. As 2011 dawned, I moved out of Anna's parents' house and back home to Bushey. My first jobs included working as a marketing assistant for an alternative therapies centre (I would sit in the spa room to work, which was great), a brief temp job as a school office administrator, and a teaching assistant in a Jewish primary school in North London.

Working with the children and supporting them with their reading and social skills was so rewarding. I worked with nine and ten-year-olds mainly, and I found that while I liked what the job entailed, it was very full-on, as I was working with four different teachers and their classes. As an assistant, you support the teachers too, so it was a fast-paced job – especially as I was doing it full-time.

It was such a good school to work in and I did think that I might go into teaching at some point. But the fact is, my anxiety began to intensify again while I was there.

My parents had been unhappy in their marriage for a number of years. I've always been sensitive to my surroundings, so I'd sensed it during my time at home, but I never knew the extend of it. They'd had a few personal issues relating to Dad's illness and it had been a stressful time for them both, with lots of tears and arguments. I tried to busy myself with my work, but it became too much for me. I couldn't cope with the job *and* what was going on at home and I was getting panic attacks before going to work. My social anxiety kicked in too, and I'd wake up with a feeling of dread and a feeling that I couldn't be around people or take public transport.

Things were financially strained. We were living on just Mum's salary, so I felt under a lot of pressure to hold down a job and hold it together. In the end, after just three months, I had to leave the job as I couldn't support the children – I was having a mini-breakdown; I was depressed and my anxiety was in overdrive. I would say that I had a mini-breakdown with heightened anxiety and depression. I just wasn't coping with my life changes, and my medication (the mood stabiliser Carbamazepine) didn't seem to be helping. It wasn't easy dealing with the end of my parents' marriage and seeing them both so hurt and upset, arguing and the fall out that ensued.

One day, after an argument with my mum about finances, things reached breaking point for my parents. Dad left the house and drove off to stay with his family. I was in shock, but I also felt like it was the right decision for them both. Deep down, I knew that they had been struggling together for a long time and that they needed to find a resolution that would work for them. If that was divorce, then so be it.

Some of Mum's oldest friends came round to support us. I had a big hug with one of my honorary uncles when he arrived. 'It will be alright Ellie,' he told me kindly as I sobbed, devastated at what was happening. 'Everything is going to be okay.'

Everyone had opinions about the separation, and even though I was twenty-three and my sister twenty-one, it was still hard for us. We wanted our parents to be happy, and they weren't making each other happy anymore. They didn't take the decision taken lightly after twenty-eight years of marriage, and it was very painful for them, but they ended up being so much happier apart.

It was complicated further by the fact we had to sell the house in Bushey that I had lived in since I was ten, where there were many wonderful childhood memories for me. The house was around the corner from my grandparents and my school. I had lived in Bushey since I was born, so leaving all my memories – my childhood home, friends, school and synagogue – felt a bit like I was being torn in half. But it had to be done.

Dad lived with us while everything was being organised, and eventually both the civil and Jewish divorce (which is a ceremony witnessed by rabbis at the London Beth Din court) came through. It was an emotional day for both of them.

Dad moved to Watford, and the rest of us went to live with Mum's sister, Michelle, who lived in Edgware, but eventually, after much searching, Mum found a flat for the three of us to live in.

In truth, my parents' divorce hit me hard. There was so much to unravel and so much had gone on that I didn't know. There are probably things I still don't know to this day, as they are very private. It was definitely the right decision for them to lead separate lives, but the changes in our living situation and family unit made my fragile mental health even worse.

I felt very low and slept a lot of the time, and my social anxiety was sky-high. Friends had to come and coax me to go out or visit them. Angry and frustrated, I knew that the divorce was making me sad, but I didn't understand why I felt quite as low as I did. I knew something wasn't right, so I asked my parents to come with me to see my psychiatrist, a lovely man called Dr P. Despite their difficulties they agreed, and Dad came with me to most of the appointments, with the agreement that Mum would come with me if I needed her.

Dr P was one of around thirteen psychiatrists I'd seen since I was fifteen (due to NHS staff changes), but he was one of the kindest and most eccentric too. He had tomes by Shakespeare and other playwrights on his bookshelf and inspirational quotes on the wall, and he was fond of bone-shaped cuff-links and wearing socks with ducks on (my dad and I had a game to see what socks he'd be wearing each week).

I was nervous when I visited his office on the first day, but I explained what was going on and how I was feeling hopeless and exhausted by life events. Dr P could see that I was finding life very difficult and that my mood had taken a downturn, to the point where I was quite depressed. My anxiety was severe, so he decided to try me on Quetiapine, a second mood stabiliser. He didn't want to up the antidepressant quite yet though, as I was already on a high dose and he didn't want to send me into a manic phase.

We also decided that I would start therapy sessions with a female psychologist, Dr T, and that I would be referred to her for CBT sessions as a way of managing my negative thoughts about life. I was apprehensive because I'd tried CBT at university and it hadn't helped my anxiety disorder, but I knew I needed to speak to a therapist and wanted to give it another try.

With his eyes twinkling and his glasses halfway down his nose, Dr P looked at me and said, 'Eleanor, I have been thinking that we should try you on Lithium, if you would like to. I know you're worried about taking it because of the side effects, but it's the gold-standard medicine for bipolar disorder. It reduces episodes and would really help you.'

I'd previously been put on Carbamazepine because I was so young, and I'd been on it for seven years. Lithium Carbonate, a natural salt, is a much stronger drug and requires tri-monthly blood tests. I was very hesitant.

'I'm really worried about going on to Lithium,' I explained. 'It's caused Dad to put so much weight on. And it's such a strong medicine – I'm concerned about the blood tests and the damage to my kidneys. Is it possible to stay on Quetiapine and my antidepressant and see if it works alongside the Carbamazepine?'

There was a short pause. 'I can understand your concerns,' Dr P said. 'We can certainly try that. What do you think, Mr Segall?'

Dad looked at me for a long moment. 'Lithium has really helped stabilise my moods,' he said. 'And although I understand Eleanor's worries, both me and Eleanor's mum think she would be better off taking Lithium. But we can't force her.'

Dr P smiled. 'Let's see if the Quetiapine holds your moods, and I will review you in a month. If we need to start you on Lithium,

Eleanor, it has to be your decision, but I will note that we've discussed it.'

The truth is, I was frightened. I was also in a bit of denial. I hadn't had a manic episode at all (not even hypomania) for seven years, but I knew that things didn't feel right. PMS turned me into a depressed, angry version of myself and I found it very hard to function. Around my period, I would get overly emotional. I'd feel low and cry a lot, and, I'll admit, I could be a little over-dramatic. Everything felt so miserable. I wasn't sure if I had premenstrual dysphoric disorder (PMDD), which is where PMS causes extreme mood swings. At that point, my GP prescribed me a contraceptive pill to try to curb the mood changes. Luckily, with the help of the hormones in the pill, I now feel a lot better when taking it, but back then I was all over the place.

I wrote a poem about my frustration with the medicine changes and not knowing what would help.

I Am a Pillbox
I am a pillbox
I diagnose myself
Mental disorder
After mental disorder
I'm bipolar, have social anxiety and PMDD
The doctors keep giving me pills
Chemicals to change
My brain and body
Into someone who can function
But I just feel like a pill swallower
An instrument for an experiment
I must speak out
Before I am consumed.

After I started on Quetiapine, I spent about twelve weeks in CBT sessions with Dr T, the psychologist. She happened to be Jewish, and so she understood the unique pressures and religious and cultural nature of our community, including the expectation to marry and have children in your early twenties, for women to run the home as well as work, and the stigma towards mental illness that existed at the time.

I would go into each weekly session and share what had happened to me that week, how the family were dealing with the divorce, and how I was coping with leaving my old life behind (not brilliantly, to be honest – I missed my home). We talked about heartbreak, the burden of having bipolar disorder at a young age and how I felt I had to be hyper-vigilant and be a "good girl" so that I didn't get manic again (no drinking or drugs).

Dr T asked me to keep thought records, in which I would challenge any negative thoughts – for example, *I can't go to the party, because I will be on show and everyone will look at me* – in the hope that it would help change my anxious thought patterns and behaviour. Unfortunately, it didn't work, because my subconscious anxiety was too strong to be combatted at times, but still, having someone to talk to and process everything was a lifeline. I will always be grateful for my sessions with Dr T, who helped me understand who I was and why I was struggling. As I hadn't been manic or hypomanic in a long time, Dr T wondered whether I had a unipolar depressive disorder (only depressive episodes, with no mania), instead, but I always knew that I didn't because my dad had been diagnosed with bipolar disorder. It was an interesting theory, though, as it had been almost ten years since I'd last had a manic episode.

It was through Dr T and an anxiety reduction exercise called the Linden method that I learnt about exposure therapy. Essentially, exposure therapy for social anxiety means exposing yourself gradually to the feared situation. Being around people and crowds was a challenge, and so I had to dip my toe in the water carefully and bring myself back to life again. Dr T worked with me to set small goals to get me out the house, such as walking down the road or going into a shop. At this time, just walking outside the house and having people see me caused me anxiety. Some weeks I could do the challenges and others I couldn't because my anxiety was too high.

In general, this wasn't an easy time for me. But I still had a goal to work towards: drama school.

CHAPTER 12

LIVING WITH SOCIAL ANXIETY

In early 2011, I decided I wanted to train to teach drama in a secondary school. I had applied to various university courses to do a postgraduate certificate in education (PGCE) and had an interview at Middlesex University. The test involved observing a drama lesson in a school and then being grilled on my theatre practice (how I teach) by the course's head lecturer. Unfortunately, despite studying drama at Goldsmiths and getting a 2:1, they felt I didn't have enough practical experience of teaching, and so my dream was put on hold.

When I received this news, I knew that I wanted to learn more about theatre and develop my own practice so that I could work with children. I'd dreamt of going to drama school since I was a little girl, so I set about researching courses for master's degrees that would deepen my knowledge. I came across a course called Applied Theatre: Drama in Education and Community at the Royal Central School of Speech and Drama, which is based in Swiss Cottage in London. Central is a famous institution, a centre of excellence for theatre, and it's now part of the University of London. It has trained many of Britain's leading actors and theatre makers, including Sir Lawrence Olivier, Dame Judi Dench, Vanessa Redgrave, Jason Isaacs and producer Cameron Mackintosh, amongst others. It's a theatre conservatoire; I wanted to be surrounded by experts in the industry and build a successful career.

The MA (Master of Arts) course in Applied Theatre would look at using theatre and drama in many different settings – schools, community spaces, prisons – and how it could be implemented to change people's lives. Having worked in a primary school, I was keen to get some more experience working with children, and the course offered placements with leading theatre makers and companies in applied settings.

First though, I had to get in! My confidence was still a little low, so I had no idea if I could be a student at this amazing conservatoire. Luckily, I still had a passion for drama and so I put together a personal statement discussing my love for theatre and my determination to teach and improve children's lives. Thankfully, I got asked to an interview for the course! I was delighted and so excited about visiting the campus.

My interview during the afternoon, and I made my way into London on the Tube. I was very nervous, but excited, and my love for theatre and desire for further study helped me through the anxiety. I was ready to take this new step.

Central is located on a quiet street in Swiss Cottage, surrounded by beautiful white houses. To get to the legendary Central steps, you have to walk down the little cul-de-sac, passing food markets, cafés and a theatre. The first time I saw these steps, I was in awe. Upon each one is written the name of a famous alumnus (usually an actor). I climbed them eagerly, spotting Dame Judi Dench's and other theatrical legends' names as I went. My heart felt warm and my tummy was filled with butterflies. *This* felt like me. Now I was going to have the identity I always wanted for myself.

As part of the interview process, we were put into groups to do a written assignment test. I cannot for the life of me remember what the question was, but I was scribbling away, hoping all my knowledge and experience would be enough! After the writing assignment, we had an interview with the head of the course, Dr Selina Busby. Selina is an expert in applied theatre in community settings and previously worked as a teacher before becoming a lecturer. With her curly blonde hair and a radiant smile, she can only be described as a bubbly ray of light. She welcomed me into her office in her calm way and we spoke about my passion for theatre. She asked me why I wanted to join the applied course and what I wanted to achieve over the year. She instantly made me feel comfortable, and that Central was the place I should be. I left feeling exhausted, but happy. I was one step closer to making my dream a reality!

I cried with joy when I was offered a place on the course a few weeks later, in April 2011. There would be lots of distractions as my parents were mid-divorce, but come September I would be focusing on my passion. I just couldn't believe I was going to be a Central student! This incredible institution for the arts had given me a place!

I wrote the following in my diary:

'The enormity of going to Central has hit me. I will (please God) be studying at one of the best drama schools in the world. I, Eleanor Segall, am going to be studying my master's degree at drama school, where I have wanted to go since age ten ... This is a huge blessing after all the adversity I have faced. I will never forget it.'

A few days after I found out that I had a place at Central, I wrote a letter to myself about what I wanted out of life.

'Dear Self,

I want a future without agoraphobia and social anxiety, where I can control it, so it doesn't become a problem in my everyday life. I want a life. I want to go out and have fun with my friends.

It's all just thoughts and my nervous system, and I can conquer it. I must think of a serene place to calm my thoughts. I must train my mind to be calm. I will train my mind.

Eleanor (16th April 2011)

*

Before my anxiety had kicked back in, I'd been in a good place with my mental health, going to parties and spending time with friends. But with everything that was going on at home – and because I'd been taking the wrong medication – my mood had taken a downturn to the point that I was cancelling social events, so getting into drama school was a definite move in the right direction. I had six months to get myself in the right headspace for it, which felt achievable, as long as I sought support.

I was scared, though, about trying to overcome what felt like an overwhelming mountain of anxiety. I was used to "blanking out" and using sleep as an escape from my painful thoughts. Ultimately, I slept too much. I often felt tearful and scared, but my friends were fantastic and most of them understood what I was going through. It really was a case of taking things hour by hour and day by day.

I was embarrassed to talk to my psychiatrist about how I was feeling. Even the thought of going outside the house paralysed me with fear, in case I saw another person. This was social anxiety at its height, and because it wasn't rational, I felt that it was *my* fault, that I myself had created the thought patterns that were making me afraid of everything.

In time, I would learn that it wasn't my fault, that this fear was a result of past trauma, being judged for my bipolar disorder, and feeling out of control at a young age. But that realisation would come later.

I tried to do small, achievable tasks to give myself a sense of accomplishment. I couldn't see friends, go for a walk, or go to job interviews, so I felt as though my life was shrinking down. It was so limiting. My GP eventually came to see me because I was too worried to leave the house. She prescribed me beta blockers to help the physical symptoms of anxiety and referred me back to psychiatry to get more support.

I journaled a lot, writing quite a revealing entry about life as a twenty-three-year-old with bipolar disorder:

If I was to describe how having bipolar disorder makes you feel, it's like having two "yous". I mainly suffer from depression, and so one "me" hides from the world, feeling frightened, anxious, down. I feel like I can't do anything – go to work, see friends, walk down a road. And the other "me" is my bubbly, happy self – seeing friends and loving theatre, music, nature, travelling and life. I am, believe it or not, a people person. But then irrationality takes over me and I don't know who I am. I become a scared child who hides in her bed for comfort. I become someone that I don't know, and I don't want this anymore.

I don't want to be so frightened. I want to live.

Part of my pain is due to a separate anxiety that bubbles up when I am under stress. I feel a sickening fear gurgling away in my stomach; my palms sweat and my mind replays the fearful scene over and over. I isolate myself because I become scared of people's judgement of me. It's irrational but the physical symptoms feel very real.

I know I can get better and rid myself of the symptoms. I know I can move forward and follow methods that will get rid of it. I just have to use all the advice to keep pushing forward. To keep challenging myself. I can do it; I can get better. I will be without anxiety for good.

What I didn't realise then is that I would always have some element of anxiety in certain situations in my life, but the key is *embrace* it rather than trying to get rid of it all the time.

Through my CBT sessions with Dr T, I started to improve, although I wasn't "cured". I also found that having my friends visit really helped my anxiety, as I felt loved and secure with them. Anna had got married in the February, and though it was a special thing to celebrate, it was a definitely a big change, and the fact that I was still single weighed on my mind. I worried about my past relationships and whether I would ever find "the one". This preoccupation was culturally based, because most of my friends got married in their early to mid-twenties. I put a lot of pressure on myself to fulfil this life dream. I hadn't achieved it, and in my mind that made me a failure.

On the other hand, my drama dream was now coming true, so I had something to focus on and aim for. There were thirty of us on our master's course, and we came from all over the world to study there, including Finland, China, USA, Greece, Germany, Italy, Norway, Poland and other countries. We would be learning about how to apply drama to different settings and go on placements tailored to our individual interests. London is a world-class city for theatre and performance, so there were hundreds of theatres and drama companies to choose from.

I'd told Selina that I wanted to work with children more, and possibly in early years too, so she organised a placement for me at a small drama arts company called Artburst. Artburst is based in Hackney, and was started by two female drama practitioners for two-to four-year-olds. It was a free programme, run as a nursery to help parents and their children in the East London area. The programme incorporated art, drama and music based around a theme, such as space or farms. The children painted, made puppets, and sang songs.

I learnt a lot from Artburst and adored going to the sessions each week, although due to my anxiety there were some weeks when I couldn't attend. My placement involved observing their programme in children's centres for kids with and without speech and language difficulties, and I found it so fascinating. The children who did have difficulties had a speech therapist sitting in in the session, helping the children to engage with what was going on.

I used what I had learnt at Artburst to create a workshop of my own, which I had to present to my peers at Central. It was based on the farm theme. I used animal puppets and pictures, story books, and a coloured parachute for the "children" to play with.

I was also helping a local drama production for primary-school children at a synagogue in Radlett. I got to work with a brilliant theatre maker in my community, and I thrived on being immersed in theatre and learning new skills.

Studying at Central was everything you would expect and want from a drama school. Central has many different courses for actors, producers, voice artists, teachers, and theatre makers of every type. You can also study the technical aspects of theatre, like lighting and costume, so there were lots of people around. In the first few weeks I developed a new social circle, including Daisy from Hertfordshire, who loved Harry Potter like me, and Jake, a community-driven person who was very interested in helping young LGBTQ people with their identities. In truth, everyone was great.

All of the students had their own talents and interests. Two of the girls had a special interest in prison theatre, and were already working with prisoners to help in their rehabilitation. One week we had Cardboard Citizens, a homeless theatre company, come in with their latest hard-hitting performance about addiction and homelessness. They were so talented! Most of the cast were homeless (or formerly homeless), and acting was therapy for them.

I was in awe of everyone I met; many were experienced theatre makers and had been practising for years. There were also mature students on our course who had been running theatre workshops in their native countries for thirty years. I was a newbie in comparison as I was fresh out of university, but it was still fascinating to learn about everyone and what they wanted to get out of the master's programme.

One of the best parts of the course happened at the start, when we took part in group workshops to get to know each other and our cultures. We all shared our stories about living in our various countries. For example, we learnt that the snow in Finland and Norway gets really bad in winter and that most people stay indoors, so entertainment is vital. It was a similar situation in parts of the USA. The Greek students told us about what it was like to live in Greece amid the financial difficulties that it was facing. I was engrossed by a chat I had with my course mate Jaya, who had been in India, creating theatre with local families. How incredible and inspiring to learn that theatre is a universal language.

I had several "I'm at drama school!" moments, including standing outside and listening to the sound of the musical theatre students singing coming through the windows. I felt like I was in *Fame*! The musical theatre students would sing at the top of their voices in the corridor as well, much to the annoyance of the lecturers, who would often shush them if they had a class going on. I remember regular emails being sent about not singing in the corridors!

My friends and I would often eat in the lunchroom between classes, but the first time we did so, I noticed a plaque on the wall which read, "Sir Lawrence Olivier performed here". Apparently, that was the room where he used to study acting and would rehearse his performances. That blew me away.

Regular alumni updates were broadcast in the downstairs café. The screens would tell us what production famous alumni – like Dame Judi Dench – would be performing in that month. Even though I wasn't studying to be an actress, it filled me with inspiration.

Making new friends, immersing myself in the course, undertaking placements and working on my essays helped me focus and helped alleviate my social anxiety. Though there were times when I had to miss lectures because I was feeling so anxious, I usually was able to get in. Everyone was so understanding and helpful, especially Selina.

Most of the course involved practical placements and assignments. I also had to do a research project, a 12,000-word dissertation on my favoured area of theatre practice. As I was thinking about going into teaching, I looked at how the drama curriculum could be adapted and made more creative for use in secondary schools. I researched and quoted thinkers of creative education, including Dorothy Heathcote, the founder of process drama (a technique of drama teaching), and Sir Ken Robinson, who supported the government's Creative Partnerships scheme to bring creators and artists into schools. I also looked into other initiatives that I thought would help shape a more progressive education system.

It took me months to research and write – the whole summer, in fact! I moved from the flat where I was living with my mum and sister to stay at Dad's in Watford. My mood was low, and I was becoming more and more depressed as my medication still wasn't correct. I was under a lot of academic pressure as well. Living at Dad's was relaxing – it was quiet so that I could focus, and he let me sleep in as long as I needed! He also understood my depression because he had been there himself.

I managed to complete the academic side of my dissertation despite struggling with my unstable mood, but it took a lot out of me, exhausting me and leaving me with a deep feeling of sadness, as though I was adrift from life and happiness. But I kept going – I had a degree to pass, after all!

CHAPTER 13

PRAYING FOR A MIRACLE

I came to the end of my year at Central in autumn 2012. I'd had the most wonderful time at drama school, although it was hard work. As well as finishing my dissertation, I had been working full-time as a teaching assistant at a London primary school, supporting an autistic child, helping them with their school work and pastoral needs. It was great, but it was a lot to deal with alongside the master's degree and I soon felt unable to cope with everything that was going on.

I needed a break.

My parents' divorce had been finalised, and I was living between my parents' houses because of my depression and anxiety. While I was living at Dad's, my mum had started going on dates with a new man, Ashley, who she had met via an online dating site for the Jewish community. Mum told us that Ashley, who was originally from Wales, was a doctor and a divorcee, and lived locally to us in Edgware. He had four grown-up children from his first marriage: three were older and one younger than me. It was still early days, but Mum told me how kind, warm and funny Ashley was, and we could see that they were forming a strong bond. Ashley even took her on a date to the Olympics to watch Usain Bolt run in the 200m final! It was good to see Mum happy and enjoying life again.

Despite this, my mood was sinking fast. I was very anxious about life and felt overwhelmed with everything. I had to leave work because I would have a panic attack before going in each morning. Negative thoughts would run through my mind and I would hyperventilate. My mind was giving up, my medicine didn't seem to be working, and I felt like I was all over the place. One minute I was happy, the next I was plunged into depression and anxiety. I spent a lot of time indoors, away from other people. I didn't know what to do or where to go in life anymore. I just slept the days away.

In the November, Ashley took Mum to Paris and proposed to her by the River Seine. They flew home and told us in person at the flat. How amazing! My sister and I were so happy for Mum, but we were also a bit shocked – they had only been dating for a few months!

So, I was excited, but still very anxious. I went to see my psychiatrist again and he prescribed me Quetiapine, a mood stabiliser that helps anxiety. I had to take it at night-time alongside my other mood stabiliser. I also agreed to start a new antidepressant called Duloxetine. Dr P explained that they would have to monitor me with the antidepressant because, if the mood-stabilising medicine didn't work alongside it, it could send me manic (although this was in very rare cases).

I prayed for these new medicines to be some kind of miracle cure. I hated living with the mood swings and unpredictability that my bipolar disorder caused. All I wanted to do was cry and sleep. I would try to distract myself by imagining myself as a character on my favourite reality TV show, *Made in Chelsea*. Those people didn't seem to have problems holding down jobs, looking good (oh for the long, swishy hair!) or finding relationships. But I did, and I felt like a misfit.

Even though I was only twenty-four, so many people around me were getting married. It was quite soul-destroying. My ex-boyfriend, Joe, now had children with his wife, and we had fallen out of touch. I'd had to let him go. My friends had set me up with someone else, but it had only lasted a few months, and that had been over for two years now. I *was* still being proactive; I'd had other blind dates too. I was also going to Jewish singles events and using online dating sites such as Jdate and J-wed, but I kept meeting the wrong men for me. Some of the men I met online lived in the USA and Israel, which complicated matters.

But then the depression hit.

I don't remember an awful lot during this time. It was stressful enough with the divorce making things hard, and then you had little old me, being hit like a train with a deep, dark depression.

As 2013 dawned, I was unemployed and having to claim Jobseeker's Allowance. I actually cried walking out of Watford Job Centre, having claimed it for the first time. I felt like a failure; my family had instilled in me a strong work ethic, now I had let them down. This was not how I thought being a twenty-four-year-old would be. I blamed myself for my situation.

Is this what my life is going to be like now? I wondered. *Will I be constantly claiming sickness benefits, unable to work?*

Obviously, a lot of these negative thoughts were due to the depression. There were days when I wouldn't leave the house, days where I couldn't even get out of bed. One day, a team psychiatrist (not Dr P) was called out to see me. My dad had called them, seriously concerned about me because I was lying in bed unwashed, sleeping from nine to five except during meals.

To his credit, Dad was amazing with me. He was still coping with the aftermath of the divorce himself, but he was a brilliant father to me. He tried to coax me out of bed with hot drinks and lunch. He would talk to me calmly and ask how I was feeling. He encouraged me to get dressed, wash my face and brush my teeth. He let me cry and spill out all my distressed emotions.

'Dad, I don't know how I can go on like this anymore,' I said, after an entire day of lying in bed. Evenings were easier for me, so I'd often join Dad by the TV or for dinner. 'I don't have a job and I don't have a boyfriend. I'll never get married … I'm on my own, and I feel so sad all the time.'

'Ellie, it's the bipolar,' he told me. 'You will get there and we are all here for you – you know that.'

'But the depression is just too much,' I responded angrily. 'It's debilitating, Dad. I need help.'

'It will be okay once we get you the right medication. I think Lithium would help you. It's helped me so much! But if you don't try it, we will have to see if the Quetiapine and Duloxetine work.'

'I don't want to be asleep all day and feeling like this,' I said, tearful.

'I can look after you at home,' he said. 'And I know you will take your medication. But if you feel suicidal, you might have to go to hospital. Keep taking your meds, and we'll get some medical advice from your doctor over the next few weeks.'

I'd had similar conversations with my mum and sister. I often phoned Mum crying and saying that I couldn't take much more. It was very tough for my family, but they knew I was struggling with a depressive phase of my bipolar disorder.

I was also dealing with suicidal ideation. I didn't want to kill myself, so those thoughts scared me, making me feel incredibly sad. I thought a lot about ending my life as a way to release myself from the mental pain, but I knew I could never do that to my loved ones.

That's when the thoughts of self-harm began.

After another long, wasted day under the duvet, I'd become seriously overwhelmed. *Where is my life going?* I'd think. *I'm never going to get better; it's going to feel like this forever*.

My pain and anger were all-encompassing, and I would get an urge to relieve it by self-harming with a razor. I thought about doing it on my arms so that people could see my pain. I'd mentioned this to my psychiatrist before, and he told me that I shouldn't do it, as it becomes addictive and hard to stop.

I needed the doctor to get me out of this deep, dark, depressive episode. Due to my bipolar 1 diagnosis, the only way I could get out of it would be to take a large dose of antidepressant (Duloxetine), engage in therapy (when I felt well enough to do so), and undertake physical methods like exercise or meditation.

We increased my dose slowly, and I started to feel a little better over the months leading up to Mum and Ashley's wedding in June 2013. Since I wasn't 100% there yet with my recovery, it was a big deal for me to be able to be bridesmaid on the day, to walk down the aisle in my purple dress and be around so many people. Chantal and I had slowly been getting to know our new stepsiblings, so it was so heartwarming to blend our families.

The only problem was that I didn't not like change. And when I am on the wrong medication, change can make things worse.

CHAPTER 14

SUCCUMBING TO MANIA

That summer, after living with Dad for almost a year, I moved back to live with Mum and Ashley in his rented property, before we all moved into a brand-new home in January 2014. This was the fourth move that I'd made in just two years, and I found it really unsettling. My mind was all over the place.

One day, I was huddling under the duvet in my new bedroom. It must have been around five o'clock in the afternoon, because Mum had just come home from work. I was very distressed, crying and telling her I didn't want to do this anymore, that the depression was so painful and I wasn't coping. She tried to reassure me, but it didn't work; I was too unwell and too overwhelmed. I went into the bathroom to get my safety razor.

Mum can't see my mental pain, so I will show her my physical pain, I thought. *I'll cut my arm. If she sees blood, she will understand.*

So, I dragged my safety razor across my arm, but it only left a small scratch with a teeny bit of blood. I didn't feel relieved at all; I just wanted my parents to see how much pain I was in. Trust me to self-harm with a razor with a safety mechanism! But obviously I'm pleased it didn't work as intended.

I showed Mum, who panicked, and as Ashley is a GP, he encouraged her to speak to my psychiatrist and let the team know what was happening. Mum and Ashley were advised to hide any sharp objects or pills while I was in this state of mind. They also gave us an emergency number for the crisis team if it was needed. Dr P advised me to continue to take my medicines, and to get in touch if anything else happened so I could get more support.

I don't share this story to advocate for self-harming behaviours, but I want to be as real as possible about what happened to me during my depressive episode. I was in a lot of emotional pain. Depression is not rational; you become a different person and your thought processes change. I never tried to self-harm again, even if I had thoughts of doing it.

I promised my family that I would tell them if I felt suicidal, and that I wouldn't act on it. I felt as though I didn't have much to live for and that the world would be better without me in it. It was only my love for my family and friends – along with their support – that stopped me from taking an overdose. It must have been devastating for Mum and Ashley to hear me say I didn't want to live anymore. I cried a lot and was incredibly frustrated.

Once the Duloxetine really started to kick in, I began to feel a little brighter. I started to sleep normal hours and was able to wash and dress. I wanted to see friends and begin filling my days with activities again. I got a job at a primary school, working as a teaching assistant in a Reception class. I started dating again, on and offline. I'd also applied to study in a seminary in Israel during the summer of 2014 to gain more religious knowledge and was making plans to live in Jerusalem. I'd had this dream for a while – I'd even started going to Jewish learning classes at the JLE (Jewish Learning Exchange) in London. In short, I was beginning to live my life again and things felt good. I couldn't believe how well the antidepressant was working! The depression was slowly lifting, and I felt great. I could live again.

Or so I thought.

Just as I was reaching this turning point, Grandma Norma became ill with end-stage Parkinson's disease, and she passed away in January 2014. Grandma and I had been close. She was a lovely, gentle lady with a kind soul. Hers was the first of all my grandparents' passings, and it was desperately sad. Our family commenced shiva week (the Jewish week of mourning) as was customary, and lots of family and friends came round to my aunt's home for prayers. It was a unique time with all the family gathered together and we ate dinner in each other's company every day.

I was so vulnerable, and my good mood was already tipping over into hypomania. I didn't realise this, though; I thought I was just feeling better and wanting to see friends, date men and go out more. I did remember the warning from Dr P that you have to be careful with antidepressants if you have bipolar disorder – as too many can make you high – but my family just didn't recognise the hypomania. After all, I hadn't had it in a decade, and I just seemed happier than normal.

It wasn't until that February that I realised that I was hypomanic, bordering on full-blown mania.

Hypomania can make you overreact and react differently to normal – for example, it can make you more irritable and angrier. I was like this with friends, family and people I dated. Basically, I was a nightmare – rude, obnoxious and arrogant – because hypomania makes you feel that you and only you are right. It was when I started arriving at work later and later each day that I felt my life was beginning to unravel.

One morning, I woke up and decided that I had to reunite my family from all over the world. I planned to create a family reunion in London for a hundred of my family members on my dad's side, who lived in America. As I excitedly got on my Tube carriage, I scribbled an elaborate family tree in my notebook. I was so engrossed that I lost track of time and didn't realise I was late for work.

Half an hour later, I looked at the family tree in my notebook and could not for the life of me understand what I was thinking. Why would I want to bring a hundred people to London? What was happening to my mind? I was clearly suffering from racing thoughts and the intense creativity of the manic phase, and that wasn't good. I felt like I was going crazy, but I carried on, not knowing that this was the start of a manic episode.

That week, I went to the theatre to see the musical adaptation of *The Bodyguard* with my Aunt Mandy. I was very excited as it was starring singer Beverley Knight and I love Whitney Houston's music. My aunt could tell straight away that something was up; I was acting like an excitable child. 'One day soon I will be on that stage – I'm destined to be a West End actress!' I declared.

I had it all planned out: I was going to give my CV to the casting director at the stage door and get a job in the ensemble (despite the fact I had never trained in musical theatre). I bought as many of the albums as I could and even got us bumped up to the stalls. I then asked Mandy if we could go to meet Beverley Knight at the door, as I had prepared a card for her saying how much I loved her and wanted to perform with her.

This was out of character for me. I am a shy person by nature and never enjoy going to stage doors or meeting celebrities, because I get nervous. That night, though, I was excitable and couldn't stop talking. My aunt waited for me and then made sure I got home safely, but then she rang my dad up, concerned that I was manic and needed treatment.

Dad was living in Brighton, as he had moved there for work. He called my mum and Ashley and asked them to keep any eye on me. Mum phoned my psychiatrist, who immediately told her to reduce my dose of the Duloxetine and stop taking it over time, as it could be making me high, and that he would monitor me. He told me to rest at home and avoid stimulation from activities and substances like caffeine.

The night after the theatre, I made my way up to the Strand after work to visit the Adelphi Theatre again, my CV in hand. This would be my big break; I was going to be a theatre star! I arrived at Charing Cross station and immediately saw a homeless man, drunk and sitting in a sleeping bag, with a pot of coins at his feet. Being disinhibited, I immediately started talking to him. I asked him why he was homeless, what made him live on the street, and did he want any food? I sat on the floor, talking to him for ten minutes about his life. He told me he had lived on the streets for thirty years, that he was an addict, and that he could do with some food and drink. That night, I decided that it would be my mission to save the homeless!

First, though, I had to revisit the Adelphi. I arrived at the stage door and chatted quite amiably with one of the admin staff about the shows and how I wanted to work there, before handing in my CV. I was probably talking quite quickly, but I made her laugh and she liked me. It was about nine o'clock at night by now, but instead of making my way home, I decided that I needed to get some food and drink for the homeless man in the station. What ensued was several hours searching for coffee shops that would give food away to the homeless.

I spoke to the staff in Pret a Manger about how I wanted to get food, not only for the man in the station, but also for every homeless person I passed in The Strand.

It was then that I had the genius idea to set up a volunteering network to deliver the food that Pret gives away every day to those on the streets. Even better, we could register it as a charity! I was going to save the homeless *and* I was going to have a brand-new career as an award-winning actress in the West End. It would be a win-win for all involved.

I eventually got the food and drink to the homeless man, but then I saw a couple sheltering in sleeping bags in the doorway of a shop. They looked cold and had nothing with them. They told me they couldn't pay their rent, so they'd come up to London to get work. They hadn't eaten dinner, so Saviour Eleanor decided to step in again.

I know, I thought. *Let's see if the Pizza Express across the street will give me some free pizza for the homeless!*

So, indefatigable and buoyed by a false confidence, I went to Pizza Express, where I managed to convince the staff to donate the last pizza of the day to the homeless couple. I also told these strangers to go to the police station and said I would transfer them some money to help keep them going. In my manic state, they weren't strangers to me – they were people I needed to save!

It must have been halfpast ten at night at this point, so I made my way home. When I got in, I told my mum that I was going to transfer money to this couple, and she looked horrified.

'Eleanor, that's *your* money,' she told me. 'You don't know these people. They might not be genuine!'

'Of course they're genuine, Mum. They're homeless!' I retorted, all the while trying to complete a bank transfer to them from my account. 'They have nothing. We *have* to help!'

When manic, people are more susceptible to spending money – or, in my case, giving it away. Mum had to physically stand over the computer to stop me doing it! Eventually, she hid my debit cards and took away my wallet. She'd only done it to protect me, but I was furious!

Mania makes me more interested in men and less able to regulate my behaviour. I become more flirtatious and gullible. I can't consent to things because my mind and libido are heightened, so I was extremely vulnerable. I had been speaking with an American man on Skype who I believed was Jewish. I'd met him via Facebook, and we spoke every day for a month. He fed me lies about being a successful businessman and sent me fake photos of him. I didn't realise that they were fake until a friend did a Google search and found they were modelling photos of someone else. He never appeared on video chat, so I only ever heard his voice. In short, I was catfished by this man.

I also got involved with someone I shouldn't have; someone I knew but was not close to. He picked me up one night to take me out, even though my family begged him not to because I couldn't consent to any sexual activity as I was so unwell. He didn't listen. He only wanted to use me for his own gain.

It's difficult for me to talk about mania and consent. What I went through that night, when he took me out in his car, was sexual assault, and it's been described by some as oral rape.

We didn't have full sex, but he asked me to perform oral sex on him, and he kept pushing my head down forcefully. I only started processing what had happened during my stay at Welwyn, and I was traumatised when I came home. I found it very hard to take my clothes off to have a shower. I still rarely talk about it and I didn't report it to the police, although I may do one day.

The bottom line is, this man knew that I couldn't consent, that I was very ill with my bipolar disorder and my mind wasn't right.

It was a very painful and emotional experience, and I struggled to get over it for years. It's important to highlight that mania can make you so vulnerable and that people can take advantage of you.

CHAPTER 15

GETTING HOSPITALISED

After the sexual assault occurred, I spiralled further into mania. I was in an agitated state, wasn't sleeping, had pressured speech (where your speech speeds up and is more pronounced), and was very anxious. I was heading towards psychosis.

It was March 2014. I had been told to get some rest at home after my attempts to save the homeless, but in truth, I was already too far gone.

I projected my fears onto my mum, claiming that she was the one who was ill and needed to be hospitalised. I tried to get out of the house to speak to my aunt, in the belief that Mum needed help, but no one listened to me. The mania made me uncharacteristically aggressive, and I shoved my mum against a wall when she wouldn't let me leave. I feel deep shame for this now as Mum was just trying to protect me, but I was incredibly unwell and had none of that insight.

Joe was back in my life at that point. He had contacted me via Facebook to tell me that he was sadly getting a divorce from his wife, and was worried for their young children. In my manic state, I told him about the assault. He was horrified and angry. He was very protective of me from then on, and was around a lot.

Joe helped me explain what I was feeling to my family. Mum and Ashley could see that I was very ill and that they needed help from a hospital or crisis service, but it was a Saturday night, so no one picked up their call. Another spanner in the works was that I wasn't registered to an Edgware GP yet, and under the Hertfordshire NHS, we couldn't access local services except by going to the Accident and Emergency (A&E) of the local hospital.

I felt very frightened and concerned about my mum and was pacing around. I didn't feel safe at home, so I ran out into the street barefoot and stood across the road by the bus stop. I called Auntie Michelle, a GP, to come and help. I told her how scared I was. She was fantastic and said she would come straight away.

Michelle stayed on the phone to the crisis team for the whole evening, but she couldn't get through either. She was also very calm with me, which helped as I was so agitated.

Here is what my dad remembers about that evening:

I got a phone call to say that Eleanor was very agitated and that I needed to come to see her. I was living in Brighton, so I drove back to see her as quickly as I could. As soon as I came through the door, she took me to one side and tried to convince me that her mum was unwell with mental health issues.

I recognised that Eleanor wasn't well. Her mum, Ashley and Michelle were there, and she kept saying, 'I'm fine; nothing's wrong me with me. Mum's ill and we need to get her to the hospital!'

We decided that the best and safest way was to play along with it, because we feared that she might not go to the hospital herself. Michelle took her upstairs to the bathroom to cool down because she was sweating profusely and hyperventilating. We got her to pack an overnight bag for "Mum".

Meanwhile, we called an ambulance and explained the situation. We told Eleanor that it was for her mum so that we could get her to leave the house.

It was important for us not to make Eleanor even more agitated and to be as calm as possible with her. Even though we did have to trick her (which we didn't feel great about), we didn't want her to have to struggle or be restrained.

Mike Segall

*

I have some memories of that night. A lot of it is etched in my psyche: sitting on the cold bathroom floor against the tiles, crying, while my aunt kindly wiped my face with a cool flannel; packing my own overnight bag in my bedroom with her, thinking it would be for my mum ... I made sure I put in some nice things for her so that she would feel comfortable in her stay.

The ambulance came, and as we were still under the "Mum being ill" ruse, my aunt drove me with her and followed the ambulance to the A&E department at Barnet Hospital, which was a twenty-minute drive from home.

I have a vague recollection of arriving at the hospital and telling everyone that my mum was really sick, and that people needed to treat her now. I was pacing around, despite having other patients staring at me and being told to sit down. *My mum needs help*, I thought. *Why isn't anyone doing anything?*

I was pacing backward and forward, sweat pouring from my brow. 'My mum is really ill with serious mental health issues,' I told the middle-aged receptionist. 'She needs to be in hospital. Please help her!' I didn't hear her reply because I went straight back to my pacing.

I was asked to go into a side room with a doctor and my family, but I didn't want to go in because I could sense that something was wrong. *Where is my mum?* I fretted. There were also two burly security men in fluorescent jackets standing at the door. Why were they there? What was going on?

I felt penned in, like a caged animal. I managed to run away through the A&E ward, chased by the security, but having them follow me around only made my distress and psychosis worse.

The doctor (who was most likely a psychiatrist or psychiatric nurse) handed me some forms to fill in, and handed over a plastic pot with a little blue tranquiliser tablet in. I was frightened, and since I didn't believe that I was the ill person, I retaliated by ripping up the forms and throwing them in the bin. I tapped the pill pot out of the doctor's hand and refused to take it. I'm normally very compliant with medical advice and medication, so this was a sad moment.

I was angry about being treated like an unwell prisoner. I told the doctor that I was leaving and made for the door, even though my family were telling me not to leave and to stay calmly in the room. I didn't listen and tried to open the door, but the security men sprang into action and formed a human chain to stop me passing. It was incredibly unsettling.

This was all wrong – and surely it had to be illegal? How could they say I was mentally ill and try to stop me moving? I was fine; it was Mum that was ill! Why was my family acting differently? Had they conspired with staff to have me sectioned?

I had a strong delusion that my kind, caring stepdad had conspired to have me locked up in a mental health hospital. In my psychosis, I believed that he must obviously want me out the way. Since my dad hadn't yet got to the hospital, he couldn't protect me from this. I was terrified.

My mum recalls:

When we arrived at A&E, the first person we saw was a junior doctor and a psychiatric nurse, who were to carry out an assessment. Eleanor kept trying to escape from the room. The nurse kept trying to calm her down, but she was so agitated that she wouldn't sit still.

Eleanor then went out of the room and, in her mania, walked through A&E, disrupting other patients' care – patients who were ill and on drips. The nurse was concerned that Eleanor was becoming a risk to herself and others, and that she could be harmed by medical instruments or other patients.

The medical team felt it was appropriate to ask security to move Eleanor to a room within A&E that had soft, low-level furniture, and to make sure she couldn't leave. It became evident that Eleanor was becoming aggressive and more agitated due to their presence. The senior nurse said this was not appropriate for the ward, and that if Eleanor could not take a tranquiliser orally, they would need to inject it for her own safety.

The nurses and on-call doctor decided they would need a certain number of people for safe restraint and discussed with me and the family what they were going to do and how it would happen. We gave our permission, which was hard for us, but the procedure needed to be done safely.

They used the correct restraint, holding Eleanor gently and talking to her kindly. They then injected her in the arm with a sedative (possibly Haloperidol, the antipsychotic drug). The nursing team waited for it to kick in before gently laying her down on the soft couch. One of the nurses waited with her until she was sleeping, and then explained that they would be calling out the main psychiatrist and members of the psychiatry team.

The staff felt that Eleanor needed a psychiatric assessment once she was calmer. This might have to involve sectioning if they found it to be in her best interests.

At about one o'clock in the morning, the on-call psychiatry team arrived. Eleanor had come round from the medication, but she was still upset and kept saying that I was ill and that they had to protect me. The team interviewed her to assess her mental state, and it became clear that due to her lack of insight and severe manic episode, she would initially need to be put under a five-day assessment, with a view to either discharge or sectioning.

The psychiatrists arranged for Eleanor to go to Albany Lodge – an assessment ward – in St Albans, but they were worried that she would become violent if she realised what was happening. They asked for me to go into the ambulance with her and told her that she was under psychiatric assessment.

Simone

'Eleanor, you are unwell and are now under assessment of the Mental Health Act, signed by the doctors you saw earlier. You are being taken to a hospital to take care of you, and your mum will come with you to settle you in.'

I sat there quietly, trying to take in the doctor's words. I was shell-shocked, but something in my subconscious knew what was happening. It wasn't Mum that was ill; it was me, and I needed treatment. It felt totally surreal, like a nightmare. I felt like I'd been in a horror film, and I was exhausted from the mania and the sedation. Yet, still in the throes of delusions from the psychosis, I turned to the ambulance driver and said, 'I will be the Nelson Mandela of the mental health world. I am going to help other patients who are locked in hospital like me. I am going to make a change and get us out!'

The driver, a kind man with twinkly eyes, smiled at me and said, 'I am sure you will.'

My mum sat next to me in the ambulance as we wound through the Hertfordshire country lanes. It was early in the morning and the sun was coming up. As we pulled into St Albans, a place I have always loved, I saw the sign to my new home for the next few weeks.

Albany Lodge.

CHAPTER 16

ENTERING ALBANY LODGE

I have been told that when I walked into Albany Lodge, I seemed much calmer, as though I was accepting what was happening to me. In truth, I didn't feel calm. I felt intensely frightened. I was convinced that I was being falsely imprisoned as part of a horrible plan, and that I wasn't actually mentally ill.

My memories of being in Albany Lodge are not great due to the severity of the mania. I do know that I was very distressed and walking up and down corridors. They showed me into my spacious side room and my mum helped me to unpack. The unit housed around thirty very ill people with varying conditions. It was a mixed-sex assessment ward, with a psychiatry team and nurses monitoring our every move.

All of us were detained due to mental illness. I was terrified, as I still thought that I had been deliberately and wrongly locked up. My fears increased the longer I stayed there. I honestly think that being in this assessment unit was probably the hardest time for me.

On the first night, I talked to some of the other women in the garden, and we got on well. The evening ended with us drinking hot chocolate and eating toast. *Well, at least I have friends here now!* I thought.

As I was still manic and my libido was still high, I became very flirty with some of the men on the ward. This meant that staff had to watch me like a hawk, because I was very vulnerable (as were they), and some of the attention was unwanted.

The next day, I decided that I needed to get out of the ward because I was a wrongful prisoner. I went to all the other patients, demanding that we create and sign a petition to get us out.

Some of the women took exception to this when they were ill themselves. One of them said something nasty about me being Jewish and they all laughed at me. It was then that my so-called friend from the night before turned on me, shouting and screaming at me, saying she was going to "fuck me up" if I didn't leave her alone. She was very ill too. At this point, I fled to my side room and gave up on my petition for the day – although I was still plotting my escape.

I phoned my family daily to ask them to let me out and to warn them that I had been locked up unlawfully. I wasn't sleeping or resting; I was constantly walking, sometimes barefoot, through the corridors. I would bang on the windows of the nurses' station, asking them to release me and to see my petition. I kept asking for more paper and pens to write my rants and letters to doctors.

I was out of control, irritable, aggressive, disinhibited and frenzied, as the mania took control of my brain.

I had no insight into my behaviour. One day, after a period of intense mania, staff took the decision to inject me with an antipsychotic medication for the safety of myself and others, as I refused to take an oral tranquiliser again.

This was one of the worst moments of my stay at Albany Lodge. I wasn't asked how they were going to restrain me because I was deemed not to have insight or consent. Restraint is meant to be done for the patient's best interest, but a few things happened that made this problematic for me. Firstly, the nurses took hold of either side of me and got me to go to my room. I acquiesced at this point, thinking it best to go along with it. But then I became distressed when they suggested injecting me. They asked me to lie on my bed and gently held me face-down so that I could be injected in my buttocks with an antipsychotic. I cried afterwards, and I was so exhausted that I fell asleep.

This is emotionally painful for me. I understand that I was very ill and needed to be injected with medication, but as I am a religious woman and very private about my body, being injected in my bottom crossed a line that I was not comfortable with, even in my delirious state. *Why could they not do it in my arm?* I wondered.

It might be that this was the safest way for them to do it, but because I wasn't asked and it made me feel exposed, I was intensely upset, angry, and determined to get the correct care for myself. I was also dealing with the aftermath of all that had gone on with men before I came into hospital, and the fact that there had been male nurses in the room watching as my clothes were pulled down stayed in my mind.

At this point, I was so distressed that I felt I needed an advocate outside of my family, and I contacted a mental health lawyer to represent me. I picked my lawyer from a list given to me by the nursing team as his surname sounded Jewish, which felt like the safest option.

My parents were concerned that I had asked for legal representation and my dad spoke to me about it. He also spoke to the lawyer concerned and reiterated that I wasn't in my right mind. However, I was entitled to have representation under law.

I spoke to the lawyer on the phone and we arranged to meet at the unit. He listened to me when I asked if he could instruct the nursing team to only inject me in my arm, and immediately wrote a legal letter to them saying that "his client had requested not to be injected in the buttocks but only the arm". This was fantastic for me and helped me maintain a sense of control in a frightening situation.

However, I didn't stop there. I wanted to go to a tribunal to overturn my section. My parents were upset that I would be going through the whole legal process, especially as I wasn't in my right mind. They were worried it would distress me further, but due to the law, I could instruct a lawyer even though I had no insight into my own health at the time and had lost touch with reality.

A day or two after being injected with Haloperidol at the unit, my behaviour became too unmanageable. And so the day came for me to be moved to a new hospital in Hertfordshire.

CHAPTER 17

QE2: MY TIME IN HOSPITAL

I have no memory of being moved to the Queen Elizabeth II hospital in Welwyn. The medical team decided that a female-only ward would be safer for me because I was at risk while manic. But this turned out to be a blessing in disguise.

The new ward felt safer over time. At first, I was still my manic, disruptive self, and the psychosis was worsening. My delusions about being a wrongful prisoner in hospital got worse. I now believed I had been kidnapped by a criminal gang who were holding me hostage, and that the hospital alarms were really cameras, filming my every move. I even started talking to the cameras in the belief that I was in some kind of twisted criminal game. I thought I was being watched wherever I went.

There was a sweet, religious Jewish doctor on the ward, who did her best to make me feel comfortable. However, my delusions made me think that she was a "fake Jew" and I became frightened, accusing her of being part of the gang. My medical notes also state that I had an assessment with a Sikh doctor (possibly another psychiatrist) and that due to my illness, I had accused him of being a "fake Sikh". I genuinely thought that everyone around me was acting and that I was in a fabricated hospital. To me, this was not the NHS – this was a criminal place. The worst part was that I still strongly believed I was in danger from my stepdad. I thought that he was the one orchestrating the whole thing in order to keep me locked up.

These thoughts sound ridiculous, don't they? But that's what happens when bipolar psychosis gets out of control.

I was afraid of the nurses at first. There were twenty or so women on the ward and we would have to line up to take our medication, often twice a day. I got very stressed with one nurse who tried to give me a cup of water to take my medicines. I didn't want to take my medication, so I threw the cup of water at her in a bid to be free of the "criminal gang" I thought were trying to control me.

I think this situation was the only time on the ward that I was restrained and injected with Haloperidol in my arm. It was done in a gentle, kind way and was not distressing for me. It was definitely in my best interests to have it because the mania was at its height. As I got better over those few months, I began to take Haloperidol orally as part of my medicine regime, so I didn't need to be restrained or injected again (which was a great relief).

My psychiatrist at Welwyn was Dr M. She was a young, beautiful Russian lady, and as such, I was convinced that she was head of the criminal gang. The poor woman was only trying to do her job, and there I was, irritable, angry, pacing and disinhibited. It would come as no surprise to her that I disliked her intensely at the beginning – largely because I didn't believe she was a real psychiatrist. I was fed up with being ill and just wanted it all to go away.

I had regular meetings with Dr M about my fears and how I felt living on the ward. She slowly introduced the Haloperidol tablets in a bid to get rid of the psychosis, and she also prescribed strong tranquilisers (Diazepam) to slow down my system.

Dr M tried her best to keep me calm and to bring me down from the manic state. My parents attended several medical reviews with me and they thought she was very professional, easy to talk to and approachable. When they worried that I might not recover, it was Dr M who told them that my mania could not last forever and would naturally fall. She also told them she could help control it via medication; she wanted to start me on Lithium therapy, but needed my consent. My family needed to be patient, she said. We were in for a long journey, but ultimately, she believed in my recovery – and eventually, I grew to believe in her.

My tribunal hearing was scheduled for not long after I'd arrived at Welwyn. My medical team didn't think it was appropriate for me to do it, but they had to comply with the law. And they realised that as soon as the judge saw what state I was in, the hearing would be adjourned. I was challenging being under a "section 2" (a twenty-eight-day assessment hold in hospital), which I had been put under on my discharge from Albany Lodge.

At this point, and for a reason I cannot fathom (bearing in mind my mental state), I sacked my lawyer. I think he must have annoyed me, so I phoned him to tell him that he was dismissed. Regardless, it was his duty to represent me at the tribunal hearing, so he came along on the day.

The hearing was held in a room at the hospital. My parents were also in attendance. Mum told me that I strode into the room, looking agitated. The judge spoke to me and asked me why I was there, but instead of telling them I was there to challenge my section, I launched into a piece of musical theatre!

Let me give you some background here. A few weeks before I became manic, I'd gone to see the musical *Wicked* with my family for the third time. It's based on the characters from *The Wizard of Oz* and tells the story of how the Wicked Witch of the West is not evil after all. In *Wicked*, she is known as Elphaba. She is seen as a bit of an outcast and is laughed at for being green. Part of me must have felt especially connected to Elphaba as I, too, felt different due to my bipolar disorder. I loved all of the characters though, and I especially loved the soundtrack. I could often be found singing 'Defying Gravity'!

So, going back to the tribunal hearing, when the judge asked me why I was there, I began pacing around the room. 'I'm Elphaba;

I'm the same as the green witch!' I declared, before launching into the lyrics from 'Defying Gravity', singing you can't hold me down. I sang. I was probably trying to communicate that I was unwell and that I would escape from all the people trying to hold me back, just like Elphaba escapes from her captors. Only I could turn this into something theatrical!

I clearly wasn't capable of rational thought or providing evidence, and although my lawyer spoke for me, the judge dismissed the case within a matter of minutes. He could see that I was too ill to leave hospital.

I can now look back with a smile at what I call my "Elphaba moment", but it was very distressing for me. When the judge dismissed my case and the nurses led me back the ward, I was terrified. I started jumping up and down, screaming, 'Mummy, please don't let them take me!' I cried and shouted and Mum cried too. It was so painful for us to be separated again, but Mum knew I needed treatment to get better.

During this struggle, I landed awkwardly on my foot and caused an oedema swelling on my ankle, which needed to be scanned. I was fine, but it just added to that traumatic day.

During this period, I became a prolific letter-writer to the ever-patient hospital matron, Nigel. Writing out my frustrations about being in hospital seemed to help. I complained a lot about being there, both in letter form and by phone to PALS (the NHS Patient Advice and Liaison Service). Nigel dealt with it all with incredible patience and kindness and he became my ally on the ward once I was well again.

Despite a very difficult beginning to my stay at Welwyn Ward, I did have many good times too. My psychosis started to recede over a period of about a month, so I calmed down a lot and was able to attend therapy groups and make friends on the ward. Friends and family came to see me, bringing cards, flowers, homemade cakes and soft toys. I was truly loved, and it showed. It turned my little side room into a home away from home. It might sound cheesy, but it's true!

My best friends had come to see me, which was really tough for them as I was mid-psychosis. Anna was wearing a jumper with a horse's head on it when she entered the ward, which I took as a sign that she was part of the mafia! My friends had to learn that psychosis makes you read into everything! Luckily, they were there for me despite it all. I am forever grateful for their support during this dark time.

It is impossible to mention my hospital stay without talking about Joe. Since he had come back into my life, he had become the person I trusted when life got dark. All my previous hopes of us being together had been rekindled. In reality, I was extremely unwell, and he was going through a divorce at just twenty-five years old. Essentially, we clung to each other at the lowest time in both our lives.

Joe was an immense source of strength to me while I was in hospital. He travelled to the ward to say the Shabbat prayers over food for me, and he would eat meals with me in a side room when I felt lonely and despondent. He made me smile and joke. We talked about family and what had happened in our lives over the past few years. I mentioned to him that I was praying to God constantly on the ward, so one day he brought me a Tehillim book. Tehillim is the Hebrew Book of Psalms written by King David. It's a book of prayers and it can be of great comfort to those who are ill or in despair. Personally, I found it so healing to pray, and I used my prayer book all the time.

I found it particularly hard to be away from home and because I was in a hospital outside London that was not in a traditionally Jewish area. I didn't have full access to kosher hospital food at first, and it was very upsetting. We put in a complaint because keeping kosher – the Jewish dietary law – is integral to our faith. I couldn't eat pork or non-kosher meat (so any meat) and I also couldn't eat meals that contained both meat and dairy ingredients such as spaghetti bolognaise with cheese. I got by by eating the vegetarian food on the ward at first, but it was hugely unsettling for me to know I wasn't keeping my faith fully. My mum cooked for me and brought me meals, and my stepdad went to local shops to buy me kosher hot meals. He was later reimbursed by the Trust. This was a serious failing by the hospital though, and my family had to complain on my behalf. Because I was manic, everything seemed much worse, and I felt like I was a long way from home.

Thankfully I was well supported by the local Jewish community. Every Friday the rabbi in Welwyn would bring me warm chicken soup made by his wife, to give me a comforting taste of home for the Jewish Sabbath (Shabbat). My friends lit candles and prayed for me, and many baked cakes and brought me snacks. One friend even put a note in the holy Western Wall in Jerusalem for my recovery (it is said that it's the closest place to God). Another friend who was visiting from Israel brought me a traditional cheesecake on the Jewish festival of Shavuot. My childhood rabbi, Rabbi Salasnik, also came to see how I was. These acts of kindness have stayed with me.

As I recovered, Dr M allowed certain people – including my mum, dad and sister – to take me out of the ward on day trips. When she asked if there was anyone else I'd like to accompany me, I asked if she would authorise Joe. Joe accompanied me on several trips off the ward, including to Stanborough Lakes, a beautiful park near the hospital.

On one warm summer's day, we sat on the grass and talked about our lives and what the future held for us. We ate ice cream and joked around a bit about our past. Joe was feeling quite low and depressed about his life. I wanted to take his pain away, but I couldn't. He was worried for his children and was grieving the end of his marriage.

'I hope things get easier for you,' I told him, giving him a hug.

'You too,' he smiled at me slightly, but I could see such sadness in his eyes.

I didn't know what to think now that Joe was back in my life. All I knew was that he was here now and that he wanted to help me get better. Joe had seen a lot of painful things that had happened to me and there was real love for him in my heart. But the circumstances were nightmarish for us both, and it just wasn't the right time for either of us to embark on any kind of relationship.

Dr M had said that I could be discharged in the April, as I was improving and was begging her to let me leave. And so I went home, still feeling partly manic, and for that reason I don't have any recollection of it. I was under the care of the crisis team, with psychiatric nurses visiting me at home every day. Unfortunately, because I was still manic, I forgot to take the right dosages of my medication and wouldn't let my parents help me.

I was rapidly spiralling out of control again. I forgot to take some of medication completely because my thoughts were racing too much. I was fearful of being at home and angry at the world; the delusion that I had been locked up in hospital by my stepdad overwhelmed me again and I feared for my life.

On one occasion, the crisis team came to see me. I refused to let Mum and Ashley speak to them because I was convinced they were dangerous and that I would end up back in hospital due to their "lies". The only person I trusted was Joe, who had been visiting me at home. He became my backbone and he would sit with me in meetings with the crisis team to support me.

For some reason, the crisis team didn't pick up on the fact that my psychosis had worsened or that I was more manic. Thankfully, Ashley told Mum to check my pills while I was in my meeting to see if I had been taking them. They realised that I hadn't taken half of my medication. It was then that things got even more out of control.

I refused to let Mum and Ashley speak to the crisis team before they left. I was riled up again and frightened. Joe tried to reason with me, telling me that Mum and Ashley cared about me, that what I was feeling wasn't real. I became even more scared that the person I trusted was siding with my supposed enemies. I knew I needed to escape these people who wanted me to be in hospital, so I ran. And ran. And ran. Out I went, through the front door, down the adjacent road, away from the house and to a place of "safety".

Joe came running after me and gently tried to talk me back into going home, but I refused to go. Instead, I told him where I was going, and I ran to my friend Nina's house down the road. I asked him not to tell my family. I was petrified and fearing for my life.

When my friend answered the door, I begged her, 'I am not safe at home. I just ran away; please let me in.'

To her credit, Nina remained calm and let me sit down on her leather couch with a glass of water. A little while later, there was a knock on the door and Joe came in. I asked them to close the curtains so I couldn't be found.

'Ellie, please come home,' Joe pleaded, but I refused, getting worked up again.

'Just relax,' Nina said. 'You can stay with me if you need to, but you at least need to tell your mum where you are.'

After a few moments, I nodded. It seemed that at least part of me knew that she needed to know I was safe.

'Mum,' I said, when she picked up the phone. 'I'm at Nina's house. But you can't tell anyone because they'll come after me. Meet me in the morning on the corner.'

'Ellie,' Mum said, sounding terrified. 'Please come home if you can. If not, stay there and get some sleep. I'll be there in the morning.'

The next morning, Mum picked me up and drove me straight to the Acute Day Treatment Unit (ADTU) at Watford hospital, as she had arranged with the staff for them to assess me.

I strode into ADTU and told the staff that I was being abused. They knew my history and could see how ill I was, so (to their absolute credit) they took instant action and led me to a side room, away from the other patients in the unit. What I didn't know, though, was that this was the room for people who need hospitalisation to keep them safe.

Meanwhile, my mum and dad were beckoned to go down a corridor and into another room. No one would let me in. They were talking to my psychiatrist, Dr R, and telling him what had been happening. They told him all about my delusions and running away from home and how I hadn't taken my medication. Together they decided that it would be safer for me to go back to QEII hospital and have a longer stay on the unit, in order to stabilise me.

There is nothing wrong with me, I thought. *Why do I keep being taken back to hospital?*

I was really, *really* angry with my parents. How could they agree for me to get sent back to hospital like this? Didn't they know that I wasn't ill?

I completely lost it when my dad drove me back to hospital. I screamed and shook in the back of the car. I couldn't believe I was going back into hospital, despite the fact that I'd agreed to come back as a voluntary patient this time. I didn't want to be sectioned again.

I sobbed as the familiar hospital building came into view. I didn't want to lose my freedom and autonomy; I wanted to be at home. I just didn't realise how unwell I actually was and that everyone had a duty of care to get me well, even if it meant going back to the ward.

At the start of my second stay back in hospital, I was put back in a side room. My delusions were strong and I felt unsettled. I hated having to wait for the nurses to unlock the showers for us to have a wash in the morning. I hated being locked in the ward and not having the freedom to have my phone on me all the time. I was convinced that I was being watched wherever I went, and still thought that the hospital alarms were cameras.

Over time, my psychiatrist prescribed me antipsychotic medications, and the nurses made sure I took them on time. As I got more cooperative, I was able to have friendships with the other women on the ward, and this is what helped me the most.

We were a bunch of women who had been thrown together in some of the worst circumstances possible in life. Some of us had psychosis or heard voices, some were depressed and wanting to self-harm, and others were highly anxious or struggling with addictions or other serious mental illnesses. Some of the women had attempted suicide and had ended up on the ward as a result. I remember one nice lady calmly explaining that her wrist was bandaged because she had tried to take her own life. She was going to be given supported housing to help her. I hope she is well now.

Despite our ages ranging between eighteen to sixty-five – and that we were of different races and backgrounds – all of us were struggling with severe mental illness. I generally got on with everyone, but there was a group of us who formed a close bond.

There was Kaya, who was an incredible gymnast and was recovering from a depressive bipolar episode. She loved fashion, glamour and showing off her cartwheels in the corridors, and always put a smile on our faces.

We also became friendly with a woman in her late forties called Veronica. Veronica was a hairdresser and she did our hair for us. It became a ritual and survival technique on the ward. In many ways, Veronica doing our hair was its own type of therapy; being locked in on a hospital ward and away from life can be quite miserable, but us girls bonded through making ourselves feel good. The nurses let us use a side room as a hair salon, and they supervised while we shared hairdryers, straighteners, hair grips and bobbles. Through the act of hairstyling, we started to piece ourselves together again. Of course, only those of us who were recovered enough to use hair instruments were allowed to use them, but we truly loved transforming our ward into a salon. It made things that bit more bearable.

My closest friend at Welwyn, with whom I'm still friends today, was Sammy. The two of us were in recovery at the same time and we started chatting and bonding. Sammy was in hospital due to a sudden severe episode of postnatal depression. We didn't really mix much at first because we were both put in side rooms. The side rooms were dedicated to people who were just coming into the ward and who were often very unwell. These days, mental health hospitals generally provide individual rooms to everyone, but five years ago there were still shared rooms. But as we got better, we would see each other more – in the queue to take our meds, at lunch and dinner in the canteen room, and in therapy groups.

We bonded over our love of nineties music (she's a huge Take That and Spice Girls fan) and we both loved all things girly. Sammy was part of the hair crew, so we would do each other's hair and paint our nails. Slowly, slowly, we began to confide in one another about our lives. Sammy is married and a little older than me. Her little boy was just two or three years old, and it was horrible for her to be separated from him and her husband. They had only been married a few years, and she was only around thirty. I was twenty-five and single, but we connected so well.

We became closer when the nurses decided that I was well enough to move into a shared room with Sammy and two sweet, elderly women.

We were lucky that our room, which had four beds and cubicles with curtains, was quite calm – or as calm as it can be on a mental health ward – as many of us were feeling a lot better. I took the bed next to Sammy, and we shared a mirror, a sink with toiletries, and some chests of drawers. We both decorated our hospital whiteboards too.

Sammy and I were there for each other during the dark times. When things got too much, we had chill-out time and would regularly sit there with our mindfulness colouring books, scribbling away. We found it so relaxing and calming amid the chaos of the hospital. Of course, we would rest or sleep and give each other space when needed. I was scared about the future and Sammy reassured me. She was and is the most incredible friend and I owe her a huge debt of gratitude. Sammy, like me, has recovered and has not been in hospital or severely unwell since. I am so proud of her and all she has achieved through such a challenging part of her life. She was my light in the darkness, and her support got me through my stay in hospital.

Soon I was well enough to undertake more occupational therapy and join in with general therapeutic groups. We had a brilliant activity worker, Molly, whose role it was to get us to socialise and have fun. Sometimes, we got to choose our favourite songs on YouTube and sing and dance together. We had groups with her and the occupational therapists, where we would paint each other's nails. It was the role of the occupational therapy team to help us find meaning in life again, and they were truly outstanding.

One of my favourite activities was smoothie making, which we would do at breakfast time with berries, water and milk. It was refreshing to have a nice drink in the morning. Gardening group was great too. We weren't allowed off the ward very often for our own safety, but we could go with a therapist and plant some new flowers or do some weeding in the hospital's beautiful garden. It was May/June-time by now, so it was lovely and sunny. It was so therapeutic to be outside, breathing fresh air with my friends. Nature truly has the power to heal.

I also found it healing to make artwork and collages from magazines, with lots of glitter and recovery-focused messages. I enjoyed painting and found that being mindful helped to control my anxiety about being on the ward.

It was a strange kind of existence. We patients became like a strange kind of dysfunctional family along with the staff. We would all sit in the TV lounge watching *Britain's Got Talent*, doing our hair before settling into bed under our green hospital blankets. We'd take our medication, attend therapy groups, and deal with the new people coming to the ward who were very ill, all the while trying to recover ourselves.

Dr M was instrumental to my stay in hospital and my recovery. She recognised that my type of bipolar disorder can be treated with medication and therapy. She had seen people come into the ward feeling as ill as I was – and recover again.

As I became more lucid, Dr M and I developed a kind of friendship (as you do with mental health professionals). I recognised that I had been angry and nasty to her while I was ill, and I apologised during one of our sessions. She told me I didn't need to say sorry; that I had just been unwell for many months and it was her role to help me recover from my manic episode. She knew that the manic-presenting person was not the true me. She separated the real Eleanor from the bipolar disorder and saw a desperately ill twenty-five-year-old with hopes and dreams for the future. Her kind heart and incredible aptitude for her job meant that I recovered much better than I might have done with someone else. Dr M in many ways helped save my life, and I am so grateful for that.

After a few months, I felt better enough to go home. To prepare me for discharge, I attended some therapy groups in the day unit at Welwyn, helpful subjects such as art therapy and relaxation. It wasn't nice to leave the nurses, occupational therapists, and Molly, our activity worker. My personal therapist, Katherine, oversaw my general care plan and helped me with a plan for what I could do upon coming home, including things like activities and tasks to help my anxiety. These involved taking public transport, going to synagogue and (eventually) getting back to work.

I cried when I had to leave in June 2014. I wanted to go home, but I didn't want to leave behind Sammy and all that I had known there.

What I hadn't prepared for was just how hard coming home from hospital would be.

CHAPTER 18

RECOVERING IN THE COMMUNITY

In truth, although I had recovered significantly, I was traumatised when I came home from the inpatient ward. This wasn't the fault of the brilliant staff who got me well – I had good treatment – but a result of the trauma of going into sudden psychosis, arriving at A&E when I didn't understand what was happening to me, my lack of insight into my illness, and some experiences with other patients in hospital.

Even though I've described the good times that I had with my incredible new friends, acute mental illness wards are not all lovely, harmonious places to live. Everyone is there because they're seriously ill with one of a variety of mental illnesses. People tried to self-harm; others had panic attacks, and some were quite aggressive.

There was a woman on the ward who I think had schizophrenia and a drug addiction. She was usually friendly and calm, but one day she took a disliking to me. I don't know if she saw me as an easy target, but she became quite violent towards me. I was the last person leaving a group therapy session, and, entirely unprovoked, she grabbed me from behind and tried to hold me in a headlock. I screamed, trying to twist myself away and overpower her. Thankfully, staff and other patients heard and released me. It was terrifying! I ran into my side room and locked the door – something I did a lot if someone was kicking off at the staff. The same woman also shoved a heavy cleaning trolley at my leg, leaving bruises. Luckily, this intimidation didn't last very long and she apologised, but it was still seriously scary. Later, we realised that someone from outside had given her illegal drugs.

I once walked in on another service user self-harming with a piece of wood that they'd managed to break off their cupboard, bashing it on their own head. I quickly alerted the nurses, who went to help the patient. There was a lot of screaming and crying. I heard things like this almost every day on the ward.

We would hear the screams of new patients who were coming to the ward for the first time. They usually arrived at around one or two o'clock in the morning and were often very ill, angry and confused. One night, I woke up to the sound of a new person swearing and screaming at the top of her voice. The emergency alarms were going off (they would activate whenever staff needed people from other wards to come and help). The doors to our rooms were always open as we needed constant observation, so it was impossible not to hear it. The noise went on and on for about ten to fifteen minutes. It was horrible.

This all meant that I arrived home an absolute nervous wreck. I was, in short, a broken woman. I have never experienced anxiety like it and hope I never will again. I couldn't sit still and the only thing that would calm me down was colouring in patterns in my book. I would sit there for hours feeling pumped with adrenaline, my heart beating very quickly, worrying about how I would fill my time because I was too ill to go back to work.

I was totally institutionalised. I wanted to eat my meals at the same time (in hospital, dinner had usually been at about halfpast five or six o'clock) and know where all of my property was at any given time (because things could get stolen or go missing in hospital). I felt unsafe in my own home because I'd been sexually assaulted. I began to project my fear, thinking that the man who assaulted me was tracking me down, so I withdrew into myself and decided to turn my phone off (after I had blocked his number). I didn't speak to my friends or family on the phone for several weeks. I had no confidence and was a shell of a person.

But there was a light on the horizon.

Dr M had not been able to start me on Lithium (a mood stabiliser) in hospital as it was too complicated, so in my handover meeting from hospital, she passed me over to my new psychiatrist, Dr R, and his team of occupational therapists and nurses. Apparently, I would benefit from a special unit at Watford General Hospital called the Acute Day Treatment Unit (ADTU). This was a unit that most people went to in order to avoid an acute hospital ward, but I would be sent there as part of my recovery.

Bearing in mind that I didn't want to leave the house or interact with anyone, starting at ADTU was a challenge. I felt so anxious about having to go to the unit on a daily basis, and I was distressed in general – I had left a hospital ward only to mix with more ill people! Not only that, but I had previously had a false start at the ADTU when I left hospital the first time, and I was still very manic, so I was terrified of what the staff would think of me.

The ADTU is a monitoring and recovery unit for people who are struggling with their mental health or who have come out of hospital. We were encouraged to go five times a week at the beginning, and at the weekend if we needed it. It runs two or three different therapeutic groups a day, and there would often be a targeted therapy group tackling things such as anxiety management, sleep hygiene, assertiveness and confidence-building. There was also a reflective recovery group, where we reflected on our week and what had triggered us. We looked at positive affirmations and did a "check in" worksheet to see how we were feeling at the start of our time there.

As well as the daily therapy groups, we also had my favourite group of the day: relaxation. The aim of relaxation group was to teach us how to relax our bodies and minds while in group, but also to take forward into our own spare time.

We would sit in the darkened room – sometimes there were

only four people, but there could be up to about twelve – on our own reclining chairs. The therapist leading the relaxation session would often read a script or lead meditation to calming music. Sometimes this would help us to imagine a relaxing or peaceful place and give us some respite, but often it would involve progressive muscle relaxation (where you gradually relax muscles in your body). They gave me time out from the day just to be. Occasionally, the stillness of relaxation did bring up uncomfortable or sad thoughts for people, and I found it hard to settle at first. But as I practised it over time, I would feel sleepy and rejuvenated at the end.

Sometimes, when we had a break at ADTU, we would go in the art room and do some drawing or colouring. Art therapy really helped my anxiety levels by focusing on the page and image. There were other fun, structured groups too, such as card making, table tennis or darts, along with creative writing and quiz groups. I am such a quiz geek as my general knowledge isn't bad, so this was always my favourite! We also had a shared lounge with a TV, books and puzzles. I'd go in there in the morning to grab a cup of tea and a biscuit and have a catch-up with my friends.

It was at the ADTU that I met Rhiann, who I can honestly say was a lifesaver to me in there. Rhiann started on the same day as me and we quickly realised while chatting that we both had bipolar disorder. She was probably about eight years older than me, with kind green eyes, a warm smile and shoulder-length brown hair. She is a sweet and caring person and took me under her wing, even though she herself was struggling with her bipolar disorder and eating disorder. She had been referred to the day unit so that she didn't have to go into hospital, and she was taking Lithium to manage her moods.

We swapped hospital stories before chatting about regular things, such as our mutual love for unicorns, dogs and sweet animals. She showed me photos of her pets and her kids. I felt like an ally. On one of those first days, it was Rhiann who lifted me up when she wrote the following poem:

Believe

In

Progress

Options

Laughter

And

Recovery

She let me keep it as it meant a lot to me, and it was then that our friendship was formed.

During those first few weeks, I was fragile both at home and at the unit. I would often go to bed early (at halfpast eight or nine o'clock in the evening) as I was so exhausted from the effort it took to manage my anxiety levels and get through a day at the unit. Being around new people who were unwell was a big challenge, what with my social anxiety and the hospital-related trauma. I wanted to be invisible at the beginning, so I often hid in the side rooms (helped by staff if I was struggling) to have some quiet time.

When I started, I had an induction meeting with my new key worker, Laila, who is a mental health occupational therapist. The role of a key worker is to ensure that the service user has a safe, happy and recovery-focused stay on the unit. They are also there for safeguarding and monitoring and to provide emotional support.

The first time I met Laila, I felt instantly calm. She was wearing cream trousers and a blue and white shirt. She was only in her late twenties or thirties, and she had kind eyes and a reassuring smile. She was very calm and professional, and she was always positive towards me.

Laila ran through the rules of the unit with me (good behaviour, no drugs or alcohol, etc.), and then asked me what my goals for my recovery were. According to my bespoke care plan, my recovery goals were:

- Get better by building my confidence.
- Sort out my medication so I can be stable (try Lithium).
- Enjoy activities again.
- Learn to manage my anxiety so that it can get better.

I definitely needed to enjoy activities, because I had come down from the manic high into a depressive episode, and all I wanted to do was hide and sleep all the time. I was on edge all throughout my waking hours due to anxiety. Dealing with this was not easy at all! I really wanted to use what was on offer to help myself.

'I think those are wonderful recovery goals,' Laila told me. 'We can work on them together. I will type up a copy of your care plan and give it to you later.'

'Thank you so much ... but ... what if I don't get better?' I worried.

'You want to recover,' replied Laila calmly. 'That stands you in good stead – especially once they get your meds right. Take it day by day.'

Taking it day by day was all I could do. The team offered me several objectives for the main care plan, to help me with my recovery goals. The main aim was to lift my mood and manage my episodes by using Lithium and engaging in meaningful activity.

The plan said:

ADTU will continue to encourage Eleanor to attend ADTU and to engage in activities that are meaningful to her, with the aim of increasing her mood and enjoyment in activities.
- *Eleanor will learn and implement relaxation techniques to release tension. She will be offered relaxation group to enable her to learn and apply these techniques.*
- *Eleanor needs to manage her anxiety effectively through strategies in the anxiety management group and to implement these in day to day situations.*
- *Eleanor should develop another form of expression and participate in activities she enjoys. She should be encouraged to attend creative sessions at the unit.*

- *She should explore, develop and implement helpful ways of coping through being encouraged to attend and participate in group and individual sessions.*
- *To lift her mood, Eleanor will take her medicine as prescribed, and this will be regularly reviewed. She will be encouraged to attend therapeutic groups.*

When I arrived at the unit, my mum, dad and I had a meeting with Dr R, who was without doubt the kindest psychiatrist I had met so far. I was anxious to meet with him because I knew that something had to change in my medication regime. It was clear I was on the wrong mood stabiliser (Carbamazepine) and that, in order to be well, I had to make an important commitment and move on to Lithium treatment.

The office was in the far side of the unit, surrounded greenery and flowers. I stepped into the room and Dr R greeted us. Laila was sitting in the office with him.

'Eleanor, how are you feeling?' Dr R asked me. 'How are you finding things?'

I explained to him that my anxiety was intense, that I was scared of being manic and struggling with psychosis again, that I was sleeping a lot and wanted to hide. I also told him I was scared that I could be contacted by people I didn't want to speak to.

'I know you're worried,' he replied. 'Lithium seems to have worked for your dad, and Dr M from the hospital recommends that you take it for your bipolar disorder too. I think that, by you taking it, we can drastically improve the numbers and severity of episodes you have. We won't know how it will affect you until it's in your bloodstream though, so we will have to test your blood weekly at first to get the levels right. What do you think?'

I had a gut feeling that something needed to change, but I was scared of what that would be. I was prepared to try Lithium treatment, but I was also very nervous about doing so.

'Lithium is such a strong drug,' I said, crying. 'I'm nervous about weekly blood monitoring, but I know it's essential. Will someone come with me to have my blood tests?'

'Don't worry, Ellie,' Laila interjected. 'I or one of the other occupational therapists or nurses will come with you to get your bloods done each week.'

'Thank you,' I nodded, taking a deep breath. I knew I had no other choice but to try to get well again. This had been the worst period of illness in my life. 'I'll try it.'

Mum and Dad breathed a sigh of relief; they knew that this was an important decision that only I could make. We chatted about the different therapy groups on offer and what Laila and I had discussed in the care plan. We decided I wasn't yet ready to start counselling, but that I could go to the therapeutic groups offered by the unit. By the time we finished, I was exhausted – and ready to curl up on my bed!

Looking back, ADTU was one of the main things that assisted my recovery. Having the structure and routine was so important for me when I was still unwell, and I can't thank the people I met there enough for helping me along the way; it really built up my confidence. It was good to swap stories about our weeks and create those connections and build friendships – it made me feel less alone.

CHAPTER 19

WRITING MY DIARY

Every day at ADTU, I wrote a list of achievements, including things like contacting friends and looking after my own hygiene. I also wrote a diary, to keep track of my experiences and the challenges I faced. I used it to check in with myself and my progress.

4th July 2014

What made me feel more positive today? Knowing I am not alone, that other people find being around others hard like I do. I have gone through social anxiety before, but I can conquer it. Seeing people every day makes me happy, especially Rhiann and Laila.

8th July 2014

What made me feel positive at ADTU today? Sharing my feelings in recovery group with everyone and knowing I am not alone in my experience of recovery. There are always ups and downs. I loved doing relaxation group in the quiet and darkness today, with a guided meditation. I've been having some nice moments chatting with Rhiann and Mia. I am feeling happier.

9th July 2014

Today Dr R said that my depression is lifting. That made me feel so good! I was able to go to all of the groups and have good conversations with my friends and the staff. It was a lovely sunny day, so we all took a half-hour walk to the park in Watford, which was such a huge achievement. I haven't been able to do that for a long time! I felt well enough to call Anna for the first time in ages. This boosted my confidence so much that I went for a short walk outside the house to the tree and back – it was my first time alone outside in the local area in a month!

11th July 2014

Today we had a support group where I opened up about my lack of confidence – and everyone listened to me. I also met with Laila for a session, to chat through how I am finding everything. She is so kind and empathetic. I told her that I'm starting to feel better, but there's still a long way to go.

I had a fun day chatting with Rhiann, Mia and some of the other women and people at ADTU, and when the transport came to take me home, my driver, James, was so friendly. My social anxiety is really improving. I felt so much better that I texted Joe for the first time in months and phoned Grandma and Anna. It was so good to hear their voices and know how joyful they were about hearing from me. Joe texted back, asking how I was doing. I miss him, but it's been hard to maintain our relationship now that I'm home.

14th July 2014

Today I managed to go to all my therapy groups. I chatted with Grace and Mia and some of the new men and women that joined ADTU this week. It was good getting to know them. There are some friendly new guys. There are new people all the time, as people get referred to the unit and others are discharged by the doctor. Importantly, I also had a meeting with Dr R. We planned my Lithium intake and other meds, and I had to go to A&E for my weekly blood test this morning at nine o'clock.

I felt quite shy in A&E as there were so many people there, so many strangers. What if they could tell I had bipolar disorder or was recovering from psychosis? I felt anxious. Thankfully, my occupational therapist managed to get me through the queue quicker as my anxiety was high. I am really pleased that I got my Lithium levels tested though, so I can continue with the medication.

15th July 2014

It was an anxious day for me at ADTU. I found it so hard to focus, concentrate, sit still and be around people, but I distracted myself with good things like art and my friends. However, I felt so anxious that I needed to go into a side room to be quiet and rest. The side room is a little room away from the main areas with a green couch and cushions. Laila unlocked it for me. My heart was racing and I felt sad. Why was this happening? I wasn't sure. I felt really tearful, so I only went to relaxation group to rest, but thankfully Rhiann and Grace were around. Rhiann made me laugh, joking with me about unicorns. She really is wonderful at cheering me up.

Laila made sure I had more support today. She was so kind and came to check up on me in the side room and when I came out of group. As well as this, the other OT Jemma and Nurse Belinda said that I could talk to them at any time. They are so wonderful.

I wanted to go home but I stuck it out. When I was resting in the side room, Dr R came to see me. He said that I was probably feeling lower because the Lithium level in my blood was low; it was only at 0.4 mmol/L, so it was not effective in helping my depression yet. The average Lithium level is around 0.8 mmol/L. I was so pleased that I had a reason for why I was struggling. Dr R said that, hopefully, over time my body will get used to the Lithium and it will build up and help stabilise my moods.

I got through so many tissues, but I was able to sit through relaxation group and do some artwork (loving colouring). I also survived talking to my regular hospital transport driver, Joseph, who takes me to ADTU in the mornings and most evenings, as I felt better.

As I am still under the Edgware Crisis Team, I had a visit at home from one of the male mental health nurses to check how I am doing. I was able to talk to him about everything and felt more positive, especially when I told him there was a reason my mood was low. He was a kind man, but I hate seeing different strangers every day, and my anxiety levels rise before they come. An interesting day today.

16th July 2014

I woke up feeling really low and anxious this morning. It was a difficult day. I had a panic attack upon waking and didn't want to leave the house. I was washed and dressed by eleven o'clock in the morning. I didn't go into ADTU and I am not using my phone or the internet much; my phone is often turned off so people can't contact me. Did a CBT thought record to challenge my negative thoughts and spoke on the phone to one of the nurses at ADTU about how I am feeling. Today I did lots of word searches, walked in the garden, read and coloured for a bit – all good distractions. I also did some laundry by myself for the first time in four months, which is good news.

Today's crisis team member was female, a pretty lady called Miriam with red nail polish (I loved her nails). I told her about my day and managed to talk to her, so that was an improvement.

17th July 2014

I didn't go in to ADTU today as I had a panic attack again (negative thoughts, racing heart and shallow breathing) and have been feeling so low with the social anxiety too, but I decided to write down my feelings for Dr R so he knows what's happening.

This afternoon, Dr R phoned me and my dad. I went to Dad's to spend the day with him as I didn't want to be on my own. Dr R asked us to come in to ADTU to see him and talk to him face-to-face, so even though I was sad and nervous about going because I felt embarrassed at feeling so low, we went in to Watford. While there, I saw Rhiann and some other friends. Rhiann gave me a big hug and said she missed me.

The meeting with Dr R was good. He explained that my anxiety might be high at the moment because of everything I have been through, and I might feel that way until the Lithium begins to work. He recommended counselling at the right time. I was proud that I didn't fall apart again; I just told him what was occurring and we handled it together. My anxiety levels started to fall because I was able to go through with the meeting and he said it was normal to be anxious about still being in hospital. Seeing Dr R often cheers me up; he has such a warm way about him and he is so kind to my parents too.

21st July 2014

I woke feeling anxious but determined to go in to ADTU today. I tried to "feel the fear and do it anyway", and I made sure I got up, washed and dressed. I talked to Mum about things. I did it! I was so proud that when Joseph came to pick me up this morning, I was almost looking forward to the day, despite the need to hide.

I went outside in the hospital garden today, ate lunch and chatted with friends and some of the new people in the sunshine. I also had my awful weekly blood test (it never gets better and my anxiety is always through the roof), but I did it. Big achievement.

Another first for me today: I socialised in games group and played table tennis with friends, new people and staff. Others were playing snooker and darts, but I cannot hold a snooker cue! Mia was in the group today. It was good to see her. I also did the two other therapy groups today, including a lovely guided relaxation. Rhiann fell asleep! We did a recovery-focused group where we talked about our own illnesses and what recovery means to us.

I felt so good that I turned my phone on and am getting it repaired too. It's been a good day!

24th July 2014

I haven't gone in to ADTU the past few days as I need to have some rest time at home. I kept myself occupied and read my Harry Potter books, which are getting me through the hard times. Losing myself in Harry's adventures always helps, so I am rereading them all. Dr R told me that my Lithium level has gone up to 0.6 mmol/L, which means it's almost at the therapeutic dose.

I also faced the world today. My psychosis and mania meant I acted in ways I wouldn't normally do. I deleted any inappropriate posts and photos off my social media and phone and deleted texts, including from the man who assaulted me before I went into hospital. I deleted his number too and felt much better, like I am moving forward.

Today I spoke to a nurse from the crisis team, answered the door and let her in, even though I dislike having different nurses each day. I told her what had been happening at ADTU and how I was feeling. I also helped make dinner and answered the house phone. I am slowly becoming more independent again. Bipolar can take that away.

29th July 2014

Today I wanted to be at home and rest, as my anxiety levels are still high, but I was up and dressed by halfpast seven in the morning. I spoke to one of the therapists, Ciara, who was so kind and helpful. She recommended some walking meditations for me to do in the garden at home. We did them the other day in the hospital garden as part of mindfulness. Everyone wandered round the large, grassy space. It's a beautiful sunny day, so I am going to do it outside and be mindful of the nature around me.

6th August 2014

Back in to ADTU and stayed all day. I did all three therapy groups of the day and got a lot out of them. I played table tennis with some of the women, which was fun, although I kept having to run for the ball! There are a lot of new people now as some of my old friends have been discharged. Rhiann got better quite quickly and has left now, and it's sad not to see her every day, but we are staying in touch. Mia is still here. Grace only comes one day a week now as she doesn't need as much support. I made friends with the new people today, but I wish I didn't have to stay here this long. Everyone is being discharged except me, because of how ill I was and my Lithium treatment.

One of the groups today was confidence group, and I found it so helpful because we talked about techniques to boost confidence and low self-esteem. I was also able to beat my morning anxiety and went for my weekly blood test with a staff member. I was so proud of myself. Staff have been so lovely and fun. Jemma, the therapist, made me smile with her sunny nature and cheesy jokes.

After this point, I attended ADTU regularly for the rest of August. I was making slow but steady improvements, the Lithium level in my blood was increasing, and I was finding ways to manage my anxiety levels. I attended as many groups as I could to keep busy, but I still felt frustrated that I was there for months when others had been discharged after weeks.

Most people in ADTU were great, and we ranged in age from about eighteen to seventy. All sexes, orientations and races were there. I interacted with people I would never see normally, but we all had a shared situation: we had been floored and temporarily disabled by our mental health issues. The resilience I saw in the other service users was incredible.

CHAPTER 20

THRIVING AGAIN

For three months, I had gone to the same place every day, had clinical staff on hand to support me, and was used to the routine of group therapy and making new friends. I had been restless to leave for a long time, as the usual therapeutic time there is about two to four weeks. I had been on the unit for the longest of anyone, and it felt like it would never end. I ached to get back to normal life, but that didn't make leaving any less frightening.

On the day of my ADTU hospital discharge in September 2014, we had a meeting with my parents and my new community team at Edgware Hospital, because I was being discharged to them. It was heartbreaking to leave the people who had looked after me for three months, but I was happy to be fully in community care again. I cried as I handed over some thank-you gifts to Dr R and Laila.

Laila had been with me since I started on the day unit. She was there on Sundays when I was upset at home and needed to go and speak to her – on one occasion, my dad had driven me to Watford just to speak to her because I was miserable and needed a chat! She had provided me with some much-needed hope, and I knew I'd feel lost without her.

I met the new care coordinator, Lucinda – with whom I would be working in the short term – along with my new doctor. Care coordinators are psychiatric nurses who manage care between you, the service user and your psychiatrist, psychologist, and support worker. I worked with my new care coordinator for a few months. She would come to see me weekly to discuss how I was getting on and what I needed. I told her I wanted to get back to work but didn't feel ready yet. In truth, this whole time period was a bit of blur, as I was still quite depressed and highly anxious after all I had been through. I didn't feel hopeful about the future because my life had been ripped apart again, even though I had been taking my medication.

My first care coordinator and I got on well, but we felt that there was a limited amount that we could do together. I was nervous. I had been in the mental health system since I was fifteen, so I was used to having lots of new people around me, but I had never had care coordinators before. It's a big, scary thing when you go through mania and psychosis, when you get sectioned and must navigate your way through hospital life. So even though I was now back in community care, I still needed more support. And so we decided that I would need a new care coordinator and have more involvement from the team to assist me in my recovery.

In January 2015, my second care coordinator, Caroline, entered my life. I am so pleased she did; she was incredibly special and we hit it off from the moment we met. She was a happy, sunny presence during dark times. Originally from Zimbabwe, Caroline wore a big smile on her face. She would come to my house every week; I was so anxious that I didn't want to be seen in a hospital environment after what I had been through. She would greet me with a happy smile, and we would talk about my week, how I was feeling, and what I needed from the doctor and medical team. She listened to my fears about getting back to work, dating, weight gain on the medication, feeling different and being frightened. Because, after all, what if the Lithium stopped working?

Caroline spent weeks talking to me about my anxiety and asking if she could help, if we could meet in a coffee shop or get the bus together. At that point though, I didn't feel able to meet her like this, so she would come to the house instead.

We discussed the future and all of my fears – the way hospital had changed the way I viewed the world, the fact I still worried about meal times because in hospital it had been so regimented, and the fact that there had been issues with my food when I was there. Not only that, but I was scared to apply for jobs. I was scared to move forward.

I cried a lot, but Caroline would listen and break down the fears one by one. Often, we tackled it day by day and hour by hour. She would remind me of the need to take my recovery slowly and steadily so that I didn't relapse.

At the same time, something lovely had been happening in my family. In my last month in day hospital, my sister Chantal got engaged to her boyfriend, Josh. Josh had come into Chantal's life at a very important time, just after our parent's divorce and my mum's remarriage. He had taken her to Bath and hired out one of the Roman Baths at night-time. There, he went down on one knee to pop the question. It was such a romantic surprise proposal.

I felt ecstatic for my sister, but it was hard timing for me. I had dreamt of this for her for so long, but I was still incredibly socially anxious. I felt alone. It seemed that nothing would go right for me, but it kept going right for other people. I hated having an illness that sent me into psychosis or suicidal depression without my having much control over it, and if I am brutally honest, I was wondered if I would ever find the same happiness that my sister had. I was also concerned about being well enough to make the wedding.

I had cupcakes made with photos of Chantal and Josh on them to celebrate their engagement, but I was still not well enough to make the engagement party, as large crowds of people exacerbated my anxiety.

I decided that I needed to get myself well enough to enjoy the wedding, which would be around a year later in 2015. Over time, I began to plan lovely things, such as compiling a recipe book filled with contributions from her closest friends and family.

As my sister's maid of honour, I planned what is known in the Jewish world as "shtick", which included props and games for the wedding. There was also separated dancing (men and women dancing apart). I planned to have the bride and groom enter under arches, jump over a skipping rope and dance while everyone held a white parachute as confetti flew overheard. I have always loved doing this for friends, so I felt it was a role that I would enjoy and would give me a positive feeling.

One of the most enjoyable things to plan was Chantal's Shabbat Kallah (bridal Sabbath) on the Friday night and Saturday before her wedding. It took place at home, and her close friends came and enjoyed a traditional Friday night meal together. Blessings were said over traditional Ashkenazi-Jewish servings of chicken noodle soup with matzo balls, followed by roast chicken and potatoes. I organised the hen party, but I didn't feel well enough to attend, as it was in a bar. Getting dressed up and going to a busy bar with lots of people still filled me with fear.

Caroline and I worked together to see what could help me on the day of the wedding and beyond. She told me to lean on my support network and to tell my parents if I was struggling with the anxiety of being around all those people on the day. I still feared the judgement of others about my illness and I didn't quite know what to say to people if they asked how I was doing.

On the day of the wedding itself – 28th May 2015 – I was a bundle of nerves and excitement. However, as my sister and I began to get ready together at home, having our hair and make-up done by a friend (mine was in a half-up-half-down plait), a sense of calm fell over me. Chantal was the bride! This was my sister's day, a day of happiness. This was her time to shine. I tried to put any fears I had to the back of my mind and focused on being there for her and enjoying the celebrations.

Chantal and Josh chose to get married at Finchley United Synagogue in North London, which also has a banqueting suite. It was a sunny day, and as I got dressed in my silver maid-of-honour dress, I felt hugely excited and thankful, despite the butterflies in my stomach. I went downstairs and waited for my sister to enter in her wedding dress and veil.

She truly took my breath away. Here was my little sister, with the beautiful, red curly hair. Here was the girl with whom I had played Barbies and Polly Pockets, who went to school with me, who had endured the difficulties of having an unwell sister and father, who had suffered through my parents' divorce ... And now, here she was – a bride (or "kallah" in Hebrew). I was just bursting with pride and happiness for her.

Chantal asked me to travel in her bridal car with her, and we held hands as we were driven the short distance from our home to the synagogue. When we pulled up at the venue, my anxiety began to evaporate. This was a positive, happy day, and I wanted to celebrate.

We had such a wonderful time that day, right from the moment Chantal stepped out of the car and I held her train for her. Then there was the traditional religious Jewish Orthodox ceremony, which was filled with emotion and humour by our childhood rabbi. We smashed the glass with shouts of 'Mazal tov!' to symbolise the end of the Chuppah (marriage ceremony), and then Chantal and Josh were danced out of the room by loved ones so that they could spend some private time together before the reception. Family photos and dinner followed – and then we danced for hours.

Despite my self-consciousness, I was able to walk down the aisle for Chantal, which still remains one of my proudest moments. Until the day, I didn't know that I could do it, but once there, I knew I *wanted* to do it for my sister (and for myself). My anxiety dissipated when I knew that I could do something for someone else.

The wedding and the week that followed were times of true happiness for my family. In the week after a Jewish wedding, some people celebrate for seven days with "Sheva Brachot" (seven blessings) meals. These are essentially festive three-course meals at family or friends' homes, which honour the bride and groom and celebrate their "simcha" (joy) with others. Often there are games and sometimes they are even themed! Men also recite the seven blessings for the bride and groom in Hebrew. We had a wonderful Friday night meal at my aunt's home and many more celebrations that week. It was beautiful!

CHAPTER 21

GETTING BACK TO WORK

When I came out of hospital, I wanted to give back to my community in some way. I decided that, rather than receive presents for my twenty-seventh birthday, I would ask people to raise funds for the Jewish Association of Mental Illness ("Jami"), a mental health charity in London who were serving my community. I wanted to turn my tragedy into something positive, and the people in my life facilitated that. Incredibly, friends and family donated £1000. This was one of my biggest achievements post-hospital – it was truly humbling to watch the total creep up and up.

Caroline also helped me to make the transition back to work. I had to have an occupational health assessment to see that I was fit for work, so I had one with a psychiatrist. He asked me various questions about holding down a job, how I felt about life, whether I was experiencing anything bad with my mental health, and how it affected me day to day. I talked a little about my anxiety and about how I was having therapy and being compliant with my medication.

The doctor found me fit for work and recommended that I started on reduced hours, to build slowly over time. He said this would help ease my transition back into the workplace.

I knew that I wanted to go back to teaching as an assistant in a primary school, so I applied for several jobs in Jewish schools in London. I was invited in by one school and was interviewed by the head teacher and deputy head, who asked me to do several literacy and numeracy tests. I was really apprehensive about this because I didn't know if I was 100% well enough to hold down the job. But they then offered me it on a part-time basis. That suited me fine!

I started work in September 2015 and built a rapport with some of the staff. I got along great with my class teacher and I learnt a lot from them. I was the teaching assistant for Year 2 (children aged six and seven), and the children were, for the most part, inquisitive and adorable! I thrived on helping them learn, whether it was listening to them read, teaching them phonics, or painting in their art classes. I also spent time working with a Reception class (four and five-year-olds) and I knew that one day I wanted to be a Reception class teacher.

Unfortunately, my anxiety was still very high, and the stress of reaching targets was affected it badly. After several months there, I realised that teaching was not the right career for me.

It was a hard pill to swallow, because I dreamt of being an Early Years teacher and helping children learn. In fact, I would still love to do that one day.

Over the course of that year, I did find work in schools again as a one-to-one learning support assistant for two children with autism. But again, I realised that it wasn't to be. My anxiety kept recurring before work and I was unable to manage it. What's more, having to take lots of time off sick just wasn't fair on the teachers, let alone the children who needed my full attention.

During this time, I had another twelve-session course of CBT with an NHS psychologist. The sessions were to take place at the Dennis Scott Unit at the hospital, and I cried before I had to meet him. 'I can't go there,' I told mum tearfully. 'What if they keep me in as an inpatient?'

'Ellie, you're doing well now,' Mum reassured me. 'They won't keep you in a ward. And anyway, I'm here waiting for you.'

Jack, my psychologist, was a fairly young trainee, but he had wonderful rapport with me. He was kind and thorough. Every week I shared how my anxiety was taking over, how I needed to find ways to manage it, and how it was related to the trauma of being in hospital. Going to the sessions was tough because I was still distressed by the hospital setting, but that eased over time.

Jack and I created an action plan for the key people in my life, like Mum and Dad. That action plan would help them with my depressive and manic episodes. I told Jack my deepest fears, explaining that I was scared I'd never find a life partner who would accept the bipolar disorder. He helped me see patterns in my life and we spoke about exposure therapy for anxiety too. Jack taught me to be brave, to see how far I had come since leaving hospital. He helped me to believe in myself when I was at my lowest ebb.

It was apparent that I needed to find some work that I could do from home, something that could earn me money but was still a true passion project.

I had already started blogging online and sharing it with friends. I had started my blog, *Be Ur Own Light*, in March 2016, while I was still working in my first teaching assistant job.

I'd had my life mapped out. I had planned to use my job as a teaching assistant to springboard me into being a teacher. That was my professional life plan. What I didn't know was that my life was about to change for the better in a different – and quite a magical – way.

I have always been spiritual and believed in the universe (and God), and I truly believe I have been led to some incredible opportunities through following my heart and passion. I came across the Buddhist phrase, "Be your own light", and its self-help approach spoke to me. I literally needed to be my own light, to drag myself out of the darkness.

Back then, talking about mental illness (especially bipolar disorder), was less commonplace than it is now. My first blog post was a tester post about having social anxiety and how it was affecting my life. I shared it with a few close friends and family members, and I thought it would be a useful outlet for my feelings while also educating those around me. So, I posted those few paragraphs on WordPress and waited. I found that the more friends I shared it with, the more positive feedback I got and the more therapeutic it became. Sharing my anxiety made life more tolerable, and that is why I started my blog. I was hooked!

But I was still navigating life with high anxiety. When I got an interview for the second teaching assistant job (for the children with special needs), I posted my anxiety diary online and celebrated my achievements. At this point, just going to the interview – and being around people who would be judging me – was a massive achievement. I drafted the post in a notebook in a quirky independent coffee shop at eight o'clock in the morning, when I was trying frantically to calm my mind. Some deep breathing and writing later, I was able to get to the interview (and get the job).

I posted about how I beat my social anxiety that day, and friends texted me to say they were proud of me.

I was terrified about my blog being found at first. I had always known that if people knew the reality of my bipolar disorder and anxiety, that I could be shunned, rejected or trolled, just as I had as a teenager. The blog was initially about my journey to finding some type of recovery and living with crippling anxiety, but when friends and family took an interest in my updates, I decided to create a private Facebook group to post my blogs in so that they could follow it.

I needed to prove to myself that the trolling wasn't going to happen, and the only way I could do this was writing under pseudonyms for others.

I decided to dip my toe in the water of mental health writing, so I contacted Rethink Mental Illness, a national mental health charity, to see if I could blog for them. I was apprehensive but I pitched them several ideas in an email, including one about being Jewish and bipolar. I wrote the following in July 2016, which went online and on social media.

It's been almost thirteen years since my diagnosis, and I have been on a rollercoaster ride. I have known the depths of suicidal depression and self-harm thoughts. I have been so frightened that I couldn't leave the house and I had panic attacks daily. In 2014, I was sectioned under the Mental Health Act due to mania and psychosis (delusions that weren't real), spent four months on a psychiatric ward, then three more months in a day ward, doing group therapies with some amazingly brave people. I loved doing art therapy and other healing therapies and I was put on the right medication for the first time: Lithium.

This was extremely challenging. However, the love and outpouring from my friends and Rabbis helped me so much. Every Friday, on the Jewish Sabbath, I was brought warm chicken soup from a rabbi who hardly knew me. My childhood rabbi came to the ward to see me and talk to me, giving comfort. This was the same amazing man who visited my mum in hospital when I was born! My friends made me cakes, lit candles on the Sabbath for me with a blessing that I would get well, put my name as a prayer in the cracks of the Western Wall in Israel and prayed for me from our prayer books. I also prayed almost daily in hospital. It was a help and a saviour from being in hospital and not in my home environment. The nurses were hugely supportive and did all they could to get me well and feel safe, but I missed my home environment.

My experiences inspired me to raise money for the Jewish Association of Mental Illness (Jami). They are a small charity serving those with mental illness in the Jewish community, who needed donations. They help befriend people in hospital, run support groups and do many other wonderful things. For example. Jami is now opening a café for sufferers in North London where they can come and socialise and chat in a safe space, with people with similar worries or illnesses.

I wanted to raise money for Jami when I left hospital, and a year later, on my twenty-seventh birthday, I asked friends to donate in honour of my birthday. Amazingly, the total crept up and up until we raised almost £1000. I couldn't believe it. It was the best feeling knowing it helped others.

It means so much that friends and family would donate so much and so much kindness was sent my way.

I have had a lot of support from our community, but am not fully "out" with my illness yet, however the support from people when I was in hospital was overwhelming. There is hope, a candle of light, despite the darkness that mental illness can bring.

I was so scared when my blog was published, but I actually received the most supportive comments. The blogging editor at Rethink was a wonderful woman called Louie, and she was so patient and supportive of my work. I published the piece under the pseudonym Sarah, as I was scared about the reaction. But I got so many warm messages from fellow sufferers with bipolar disorder. They also loved the Jewish angle and the reaction was so positive that it bolstered my confidence. I even printed out some of the positive comments as a reminder to myself that my writing was making a small difference to others.

The blog for Rethink was shared by various mental health charities and people on social media, and it was viewed over 16,000 times. It felt like the biggest blessing; I owe Rethink a huge debt of gratitude for helping me boost my confidence to write. I was stunned that people wanted to hear about my life with bipolar disorder (and sometimes I still am). The most important part of writing for Rethink was what happened as a result of my article. I wrote on my own blog about it in August 2016:

The most important part for me was when a lady here in the UK reached out to me to tell me her sixteen-year-old daughter was depressed and suicidal, and that she had showed her my article to say, 'There is hope'. For me, knowing that my article can help others makes it an absolute dream come true. I was sixteen when it all started for me.

This is why I write. I write for my sixteen-year-old self, who didn't have blogs, magazines, mental health autobiographies or people in the public eye to turn to. I write for the teenagers of today and adults who have mental illness and are struggling. They may be newly diagnosed or in hospital for the fourth time. They may be in the community but not fully well yet, sitting at home and unable to work. They may have recovered. This is what motivates me to share my story.

Louie asked me to write more articles for Rethink Mental Illness and, as each one was published, my confidence continued to grow. I wrote about descending into suicidal depression and about how art therapy helped me while I was in hospital. I was still apprehensive, using pseudonyms such as Sarah and Rose. But in my heart, I knew it was only a matter of time before I went public with my real name.

The UK mental health campaign Time to Change had been on my radar for a while, as they prominently fight against stigma. From my email conversations with Louie, I realised that Time to Change is the campaign arm of Rethink Mental Illness. She put me in touch with a great editor at Time to Change and I pitched them an article with my untold story.

They had seen my Rethink articles and liked the idea, and so, in September 2016, under the pseudonym Sarah, my article 'I Cannot Imagine Having Bipolar Disorder Without A Support Network' was published under the pseudonym Sarah. I wrote at the end of the article:

My support network of family and friends has meant many positive things – I could get back to work in my own time, have financial help and emotional support. And when I felt suicidal, I had people there to talk to. I am aware how lucky I am; not everyone has this. Some people struggle far more with life. My support network has given me the freedom to not have to panic or worry hugely. I can't imagine having to go through this on my own as many others do.

I will have this condition for the rest of my life. I know how best to manage it, but there are still hard times. Either way, I will continue explaining it to people who ask, so that people can understand that you can live a full and fulfilling life with this illness – and so that stigma falls. Having bipolar disorder is not shameful.

To be recognised by such a huge platform as Time to Change as well as Rethink was just incredible. It was a real honour to write for them and my story reached thousands of people again, via social media and the personal stories section of their website. Reading the comments on how it helped others with bipolar disorder showed me again that I was right to share my story. Seeing the likes and the uplifting messages truly touched my heart.

Indeed, I was lucky enough that Time to Change had me back the following year in May 2017, talking about my descent into psychosis in my last episode. I wasn't comfortable disclosing it and it took a lot of courage to write this, even under a fake name.

I rarely talk about my psychotic state, which led me to be sectioned under the Mental Health Act. This is due to shame: I was ashamed of myself, even though it wasn't my fault. Rather, it was down to faulty brain chemistry and my medication that had stopped working. There is still a huge amount of stigma around psychosis and anything that makes you lose your sanity ... The shame of losing your mind is great, and acting out of character shatters your self-esteem.

When I left hospital, I sank into a depression due to the shame of how I acted in hospital and how my brain and its chemistry could go so catastrophically wrong. Kindness goes a long way when you are feeling ashamed. If you have a friend or family member struggling with this – be calm, show kindness, and show up for them. They need your support at what is an incredibly painful time.

This was a definite turning point. I was beginning to accept that I had been unwell and had psychosis, and that I shouldn't be ashamed. Writing was a form of therapy for me, and I found it truly healing. People seemed to want to hear my story too.

The most pivotal time for me was the period between 2016 and 2017, in terms of my writing and my acceptance of bipolar disorder within myself. I kept blogging on *Be Ur Own Light* and sharing my life, and after the success with Rethink and Time to Change, I contacted other charities such as Bipolar UK and SelfharmUK. Writing about my journey for them was such a joy. I also wrote for the wonderful online magazine *Counsellors Café* about my social anxiety (its editors, Dionne and Victoria, have always been such supporters of my work). All of these were such a privilege to write.

Around this time, I heard that Huffington Post UK were looking for free contributors to write articles on their site. This suited me well, as I was still working in primary schools and volunteering with Jami on a mental health project. I just wanted some exposure and so I sent a pitch email to the editor with links to my blogs and articles online.

The lifestyle editor accepted me as a mental health blogger in November 2016, and I wrote three pieces for the Huffington Post UK website. I wrote about the "Mental Health Wellness Checklist" (about self-care), teen mental health and staying mentally healthy during the winter. It was such a big achievement for me to see these on the Huff Post website and to have been accepted as a writer. They were the first articles under my real name and were more advice articles than personal stories. Through writing and sharing these, I got the confidence to write under my real name.

I was finally becoming the writer I wanted to be.

I knew that I was getting a good reaction to my writing and blogging, but my anxiety at work had crept up again. Leaving that job, I could now focus on writing and blogging and seeing where my career led.

CHAPTER 22

WRITING AND COMMUNITY

In 2016, the Jewish Association of Mental Illness (Jami) wanted to raise awareness of mental health within the Jewish community in the UK. As in some other communities, there had traditionally been a stigma about having mental illness, so I wanted to help change that, especially with my family's experience of bipolar disorder.

In Judaism, every Saturday is the Jewish Sabbath, which is celebrated in synagogue. Jami wanted to create a mental health awareness Shabbat, where rabbis spoke from the pulpit about mental illness alongside speakers with lived experience. The aim was to place the issue firmly at the heart of the community.

My role as a volunteer was to email all the synagogues to encourage them to take part. As more and more synagogues and communities from Scotland to Essex and Manchester to London began coming on board, we realised that we had hit on a key issue. In the first year, the Shabbat came to over eighty communities, with a specially prepared sermon by Rabbi Daniel Epstein of Southgate. Rabbi Epstein pioneered the project in his own synagogue in London in 2017 and we were so grateful that he came on board. I volunteered again in 2018, and this time, over a hundred communities joined. Jami have kept the project going, and although I no longer volunteer for it, I felt privileged to have the opportunity to break the stigma against mental ill-health in the community.

It gave me such joy that my dad and I were asked to speak at a synagogue in Belsize Park for the 2019 mental health Shabbat. I had prepared a talk but felt too nervous on the day to speak publicly. On the other hand, Dad (ever the pro speaker), spoke for us both and read my speech. I am so proud of him for this, as it had taken him over twenty years to talk openly about having bipolar disorder. We were warmly welcomed by families in the community. I hope one day that my anxiety will allow me to do public, face-to-face speaking about my journey!

But back to 2017.

My writing portfolio was expanding, and I began to write about my journey under my real name. I wrote for both the Counselling Directory and Mind – both of which have been huge supporters of my subsequent work – about being in psychosis and having bipolar disorder. What a boost! I started taking on further writing clients, including a fantastic therapist named Jessica, for whom I wrote wellbeing articles.

The Mind article helped me to build my confidence in my writing and in helping others. I felt that I needed to get my story out there. After all, sharing my darkest times had already started to help others, right?

My connection with the Counselling Directory led me to hear about a new mental health magazine called *Happiful*, a publication purely dedicated to mental health. They have interviews with celebrities, articles on different aspects of mental health and wellbeing, and real-life stories. I started chatting online to their editor and pitched my story to her. My more detailed story was still largely unpublished, so Rebecca gave me a brief and asked me to write my story from the heart. It was published in January 2018, and this was a turning point for me. There were photos of me on there and it was under my real name. It was brutally honest, frank, and above all, hopeful.

The reaction blew me away. I had feedback from both people I knew and people I didn't know. Everyone was so positive and kind about me sharing my mania with the world.

I have gone on to write various "Happiful Hacks" articles for *Happiful* on bipolar disorder and social anxiety. It is always a thrill to be published in their magazine, and the exposure they have given me has helped me meet further journalism contacts. I hope to write more for them some day.

My writing dreams were beginning to come true. One day, I was on Twitter in the January, looking at mental health writers, when I discovered a journalist by the name of Yvette Caster. Yvette worked at Metro.co.uk, the online newspaper based in London, and she had written about having bipolar disorder. She was the editor for Metro blogs (as they were called then) and in charge of finding new writers. I dropped her an inbox message, telling her that I was a mental health writer with bipolar disorder, that I wrote a blog, and that I was just being published online but had written for charities.

I didn't expect to hear back from her, but really wanted to write for Metro as I had noticed that they covered a lot about mental health. I didn't realise that a lot of this was down to Yvette's passion for breaking the stigma in the national media!

Yvette wrote back to me and said I should drop her a pitch email with some article ideas, but most of the ones I sent had already been covered. However, she took a look at my blog and had found an article I had written on it about weight gain on my bipolar medication. Yvette told me she liked my writing style and asked me to write a similar piece for her. I was over the moon, but also a little scared. I had never written for a big national online newspaper that got millions of views ...

I set about writing my article about the side effects of anti-psychotics on weight gain and interviewed several people I knew. My friend, author Jonny Benjamin MBE (we have known each other since we were fifteen through friends,) agreed to contribute a quote about his experience of taking medication for his schizoaffective disorder. My friend's sister happened to be a consultant NHS psychiatrist in London and also agreed to talk to me. I collated various case studies and stats and put it together in the way Yvette asked for.

She loved it and agreed to publish it, which was a huge relief as I was so nervous about getting it right. It was a dream come true. After pitching more articles to Yvette and her successors, I became a freelance writer for them. Nothing gave me more joy than seeing my words and case studies being put out there to help the public battle mental health stigma. The platform that Metro.co.uk gave to me has been unparalleled and sharing my articles on Twitter has helped me grow an online following there. I pitched many ideas and have now written on homelessness and mental health, my dad's story with bipolar disorder, mental health and sex, religion and mental health, Halloween and mental health and much more!

I hope to write more articles for Metro.co.uk in the future; they are an absolute trailblazer, telling untold stories and covering important topics. They took a chance on an unknown writer and allowed me to research mental health topics and case studies of new and exciting people.

I was overjoyed to meet Yvette in person at the 2018 Mind Media Awards. It was so lovely to give Yvette and Ellen – with whom she created the Mentally Yours Podcast – a big hug, to talk about how far we had all come. Receiving the email invitation for this event was one of the happiest moments of my life. When the email landed in my inbox, I had the biggest grin ever. I just couldn't believe it, and immediately called both of my parents excitedly, to tell them the happy news.

I truly felt like a mental health journalist, after all my hard work.

After writing for Metro.co.uk, it was my dream come true to write a piece about dating and mental illness for my favourite teen magazine, *Glamour* (UK). They had recently become online-only, and I got in touch with their wonderful editor Deborah via LinkedIn, who put me in touch with their online editor, Bianca.

The piece for *Glamour* was different to my Metro.co.uk feature articles. Bianca helped me shape the article, which was a storytelling piece about my journey with bipolar disorder and dating. It is one of the most personal articles I have ever written. It was a true honour to be featured and I knew my teenage self would be proud to be published in *Glamour*.

I started writing for more charities during this time, including No Panic and Stop Suicide. In the February, I wrote for the *Jewish News* about my story, which was a massive step. I had felt outcast from the community as a teenager when I was ill, and I didn't want any current teenagers to feel how I felt. The *Jewish News* team were brilliantly supportive.

My Twitter profile was growing, and through it I found opportunities to contribute articles to *Cosmopolitan* and *Elle Magazine*. I had already pitched to the *Telegraph* and to *Stella Magazine* (the Sunday weekly women's magazine) just after the Huffington Post articles were published in 2016. The editor Naomi, as well as being an accomplished journalist in her own right, was also Jewish, and so she'd connected with my story due to our shared community. She said it was a story that needed to be told. Thanks to her efforts and many rewrites to get it perfect, my article about my journey appeared online in November 2018.

Up until the *Telegraph* article, I had largely received positivity from readers. But as the *Telegraph* website is so high profile, I did experience some trolling from people who don't understand bipolar 1 disorder. They made jokes about my medication eventually "making my kidneys fail" (a potential side effect of Lithium). It was rude, painful and hurtful and just shows how far we still have to go to stop mental health stigma.

Luckily, I had a support network in my family, and they helped me deal with those kinds of comments. To me, it was inevitable that as my writing was becoming more exposed, I would also be exposed to the trolls. Thankfully, kind messages telling me that my work inspires them greatly outweigh any negative one.

The lesson here is this: words can be hurtful. Think before you write, and always be kind.

CHAPTER 23

LOOKING TO THE FUTURE

In October 2016, just as my writing career was burgeoning, I decided to try dating again. I was cautious, but I wanted life to get back on track and for blessings to manifest. I was impatient and being ill had showed me that life had been too short.

I was twenty-eight and I had been using a Jewish dating website called Saw You at Sinai, which uses real matchmakers to match men and women's profiles. I'd been using Jewish dating apps too.

This was a big decision. In the summer of 2016, Joe had left my life again and married a woman he'd been dating for about nine months. When I found out that he'd got engaged, I had mixed feelings. He had made a connection with someone else, and while that hurt, it became ever more evident that even though I loved Joe, he was only ever meant to be a friend. I couldn't allow myself to have my heart broken again and I resolved to find a man who wanted to stay in my life for good, who would be able to support me as I needed. Joe had tried, but his life circumstances meant he had to put himself and his children first. He remarried in the hope that this would be his happy ending, and it was the right decision for him. I wished him well, so it was time for me to move on now too. I was ready.

So, in the August, with the anxiety of an antelope being chased by a cheetah, I made plans to meet with Mr A. On the night of our date, I managed to calm my heart rate by breathing slowly and deeply, enough for me to put on my make-up, anyway. I straightened the frizz and put on a nice black dress.

We met for a drink, but it wasn't to be. He told our matchmaker that I wasn't right for him. Nevertheless, I was super proud that I had attended my date with Mr A, even if it hadn't worked out.

Then followed a year of going on dates with more men. I went on several dates with Mr B, a very religious but lovely man. We just weren't right for each other. Mr C, D and E followed too, but none of them were good fits.

My social anxiety was still so high, and to top it all off, I had my bipolar disorder and the fact that I'd been in hospital lurking in the background. When would I feel ready to reveal it to someone, and at what stage?

My fantastic matchmaker, Billie, did not give up. She believed that I would find love and she persevered for me, sending my dating profile to various men. The profile was in-depth, covering my life goals and values, religious levels, and aims in life. It also featured my photo. I experienced my fair share of rejections, but I did a fair bit of rejecting myself.

In September 2016, a man's profile popped into my inbox. His name was Robert Mandelstam; he was twenty-seven and from Chigwell in Essex. His broad smile intrigued me (as well as his height – I am tall for a Jewish girl) and he wrote about building a family with good values. He had also written about helping the vulnerable through his job and his passion for mental health. I was excited but cautious due to my experiences, and we arranged to meet for a date.

We met on a cold but sunny October day, at Café Nero in Edgware, near my home. We must have spoken for about three hours, and he had to go and renew his parking! He had such nice green eyes and an attractive smile. I was relieved to get a text asking me on another date, and this time we met at a cosy pub the following Saturday night.

I felt quite nervous. I had carefully applied eyeliner, washed and straightened my hair and put on a nice dress. I wanted to impress him, but I didn't know how much I should say about my life. Luckily Rob put me at ease.

We got chatting about mental health because Rob had a family member who has had mental illness. He also spoke passionately about his career, which involved helping vulnerable people with their welfare benefits. He really wanted to help people. I could see he was caring, intelligent and passionate, and it drew me in. In fact, I felt so relaxed with him that after a few hours, I opened up about my own mental health struggles. I would never normally have done this, but I could see how caring he was, and our conversation flowed. We also made each other laugh and talked about light-hearted topics too!

The date went so well that when Rob dropped me home, like a true gentleman, we were already talking about where we were going to go on our third date. As it turned out, that date would be at The View from the Shard. We watched the sun go down over London (super romantic) and then went to Reuben's Restaurant for dinner. That was when I knew. I really liked him. There was attraction there, a connection so special that I hoped he felt it too.

From there, we carried on dating and met each other's families. We had so much fun together, going to the theatre, parks, restaurants. We fell in love.

We started talking about engagement about six months in, but we both felt it was way too soon. Eighteen months after we first met, Rob proposed to me at the Shard at sunset, in recreation of our special date. We were overlooking London as he went down on one knee and asked me to marry him.

I said yes. It was the most beautiful moment.

Thankfully the moment was captured by some Australian tourists, who saw he was proposing and took photos of it as it happened.

I'll be honest now. I can't say I was too surprised about the proposal, because I had designed my engagement ring several months before. I knew it was going to happen, but I didn't know when or where.

We hugged each other, feeling emotional and on top of the world. We rang our families who shared in our joy. Leaving the Shard, we went to Reuben's Restaurant to ring more people, before we broke the news online. For several days, the congratulations came flooding in and we were surrounded with love.

Shortly after, we held drinks for friends. We then had a bigger engagement party for our family and friends with lots of food, drink and the Jewish vort ceremony. "Vort" is Yiddish for "plate", and during this ceremony we break a plate. The breaking of the plate symbolises finality, something that can't be undone, to show that the engagement is final too. Bits of plate are given to single women (and men if they want) as a good luck charm. Rob's rabbi conducted this and spoke a bit about us to our family and friends. It was such a special moment.

The day I found my sparkly lace wedding dress, I stood in the shop with Mum and Chantal. Mum cried, happy tears pouring down her face. After everything we had been through together, we were now going to experience something joyful. I'd dreamt about this day for years. By the time you read this, Rob and I will be married. Our wedding day is 11th July 2019 and we have been planning our wedding for over a year. I am so excited. I can't believe it's really happening and that I will be a "Mrs"! Rob is patient and kind, and I hope that we continue to grow in love and build our life together. He is my rock and I am grateful for him being in my life.

Sometimes I still feel like my scared sixteen-year-old self, sitting in that psychiatry room at the Priory North London, being given a diagnosis of bipolar disorder. I didn't think there would be anyone out there who would accept me for my bipolar disorder, for the ups and downs and the different brain chemistry. I have learnt that thanks to Lithium and therapy, bipolar disorder does not have to be my life. I can thrive and live in remission and I can achieve things in life.

Here's to the future. I hope that one day I can publish a mental health children's book series, and I would love to do more advocacy work in schools and universities. I am so thankful for all that has happened in my life. If you are a teenager going through mental illness, please know that you can recover. Seek support. Reach out to mental health charities and helplines. Go to your doctor and get help. Don't brush it under the carpet. An entire community of advocates is here for you.

My story does not end here, but I hope that you, my reader, have found this book helpful. In these pages I have brought my bipolar disorder to light, and I have no shame anymore. I hope it shows that with great support from medication, therapy, family and friends, you can achieve your dreams too.

Just give yourself that time and space to recover first. Then, go and take on the world.

ACKNOWLEDGEMENTS

Thank you to you, my reader, for travelling with me on this journey.

Thanks to the friends I have made in the Twitter community for embracing me with open arms. I never expected to find such a warm, supportive community! This includes Charlotte Underwood, Hope Virgo, Karen Manton, Fiona Thomas, Lucy Nichol, Hattie Gladwell, Miss Anxiety, Anneli Roberts, James Conlon, Cara Lisette, Katie Conibear, Tom at Messy4mind, Ross Clark, Steve Sharkey, Fred Gough, Paul McGregor and many others.

Thank you, Jonny Benjamin MBE, for your friendship, your support of my work and for inspiring me to become a mental health advocate. I would also like to thank his co-writer and editor, Britt Pflüger, for believing in my writing.

Thank you to Yvette Caster, Ellen Scott, Aimee Meade, Qin Xie and all at Metro.co.uk for believing in my work and commissioning my articles. You have helped me to reach more people and taught me to feature write, and for that I am ever grateful.

Thank you to Becca Thair and the team at *Happiful Magazine* for being the first to share my story and for taking a chance on an unknown writer. I can't wait to work with you more in the future!

Thanks to Bianca London and Deborah Joseph at *Glamour* for commissioning my articles about dating and being plus size. Thanks to Naomi Greenaway at the *Telegraph* for believing in my writing and for all of your support and editing over the past year.

Thank you to Olivia Blair at *Cosmopolitan* for featuring me in her articles across Hearst.

Thank you to Louie Rodrigues for commissioning me at Rethink Mental Illness, and to the editors at Time to Change, Mind, No Panic, and the Counselling Directory as well.

Thanks to the team at the *Jewish News* for your support of me and my work, especially Francine Wolficz, Jack Mendel and Richard Ferrer. Thanks also to Rabbi Ari Kayser at Aish for sharing my story in your magazines in the *Jewish Weekly*.

Thank you to Rabbi Daniel Epstein, Lisa Coffman and team for getting me involved in the mental health Shabbat and all at Jami – Laurie Rackind, Liz Jessel, Louise Palmer, Daniel Neis, Andrew Barbarash and the teams. Thanks to Belsize Square Synagogue for hosting me and Dad at the awareness Shabbat.

Thanks to all in my Facebook group, who give me reason to write my blogs.

Thank you to anyone who supported me when I was in and out of hospital – Dr Graham, Susannah, Dr Maria, Dr R, the occupational therapy team, and my nurses, Nigel, Caroline. Joe – for your support and kindness four years ago. Big thanks as well to my dear friends from hospital for standing by me.

Most importantly of all, thank you to:

Stephanie Cox and Katie Taylor, my indefatigable editors at Trigger Publishing, who have put up with my last-minute edits and generally been amazing – thank you!

Mum and Ashley: words cannot express my depth of gratitude to you.

Dad: we have been on such a journey, and I am so proud of you. Thank you for always allowing me to be me.

Chantal and Josh: thank you for your amazing support, and Chantal – thank you for our unbreakable bond as sisters.

My in-laws, Caroline, Martin and Alexander, for your unfailing love and support.

To Grandpa Harry and Grandma Miri, and remembering my dear grandparents Doreen Lorber z'l, Norma Segall z'l and Carol

Segall z'l, who would have loved this book.

Auntie Michelle and Uncle Barry, Auntie Mandy and Uncle Anthony, Auntie Angela, Uncle Alan and all my first cousins and their kids: Robert, Orli, Matti, Emily, Daniel, Madeleine, Jordan, Adina, Elliot, Riva and Menachem, Leora, Gabriel and Oliver.

All the Krotoskys and my wider stepfamily for coming into my life and filling it with sunshine.

Rabbi Meir and Judy Salasnik, Rabbi Baruch, Nechama Davis and Rabbi Johnny Solomon for your pastoral support. Brevice Azoulay for everything.

Anna, Daniel and family, Sue and David, and all the May family for your unconditional love.

To Hannah, Katie, Wooty and Charlotte for your love and support.

My teachers at Immanuel College for believing in my ability and helping me get well again.

To all my friends (there are too many to list here): thank you for standing by me through the years, for your love and kindness. You know who you are and I am so grateful.

Rob: I love you. Thank you for being my backbone and dinosaur face. For believing in me and my story, and supporting me through all the writing. I'm so happy and proud to be Mrs Mandelstam, and I can't wait for our future together!

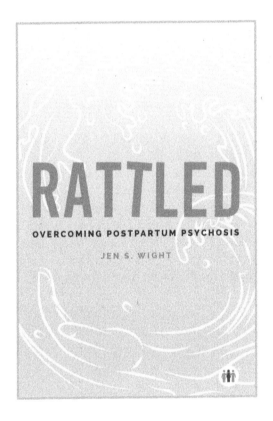

Teacup In A Storm

Finding My Psychiatrist

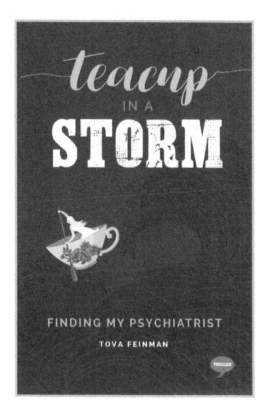

Wracked with trauma from childhood abuse, Tova sought therapy to soothe her mind. However, it was not as easy as simply finding a person to talk to ...

Burlesque or Bust

Bringing My Mental Health to Heel

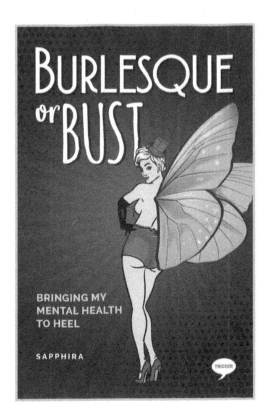

After a traumatic childhood and bipolar episode, Sapphira threw herself into burlesque dancing and was able to transform from chrysalis to beautiful butterfly – with lots of added sparkle.

EXTRACT FROM

Burlesque or Bust

My real name is Priscilla Marguerite Silcock and I was born on Tuesday 1st February 1977 to two devoted and deeply caring parents. They wanted nothing more than to support, love and nourish the precious little soul that came into their lives – this warm, pink, crying bundle of joy. I have often quizzed my mother about what time of day I was born and what she remembered about my birth. These are intricate details, some of which she has been unable to answer, because to her all that became inconsequential the moment I appeared in her arms, filling her life with light, hope and a new purpose.

My parents were God-fearing folk and born-again Christians, so reading the Bible and going to our Christian Brethren Church are some of my earliest memories.

My mother was the daughter of Second World War refugees who had fled the refugee camps of Bavaria to find a home on the sunburned shores of Australia's bountiful beauty. My Opa was Hungarian and my Oma was German. My mother was one of four siblings and the second of a pair of twins. I always loved it that my aunty and my mum looked so alike. They are both true natural beauties with sharp cheek bones and slim physiques. They are soft, beautiful, caring people.

My father was born in Portsmouth, England and he met my mother on a trip to Ontario, Canada. They lived together in England for a while, and there they got married before relocating to Melbourne when my father was twenty-eight.

We were a humble, working-class family. We've lived in two different houses in Melbourne, Victoria, in that great island known as Australia. My childhood memories are divided distinctly by these two locations, as I was just three years old when we moved to our second bigger home, the back apartment of which I am now living in as I sit here writing.

My fondest memory begins with music; my mother's voice would sing me to sleep. I could feel the vibrations of her throat as I lay warmly encased against her chest. She would stroke my face gently and repeatedly, sending me off to sleep. I know I am small in my earliest recollections, because I see myself standing in a bedroom, the bed towering above me, the boxes of toys under my bed the same height as I am.

It was in that first home I felt something so strong it still stirs within me today. It was the surprise of a gift, a small koala puzzle. I found it wrapped in white tissue paper on my pillow. The overwhelming emotion of happiness and gratitude I felt when I received that koala puzzle is still so vivid, it penetrates through the swirling archive of nostalgia in my mind, forming a crystal-clear moment in time. Considering how few lucid memories I have of that first home, it startles me that this one is so strong. I guess you could call it my first experience of true love.

My mother was, and still is, the most beautiful, self-sacrificing and caring person I have ever met. Being her daughter and having her undivided attention was simply sublime. I revelled in her tender loving care and flourished under her nurturing hands. Her unconditional love is another reason I am here on this planet today. It's the reason I'm able to write this story.

My father was a disciplined and hardworking man. He was sometimes stern and highly intelligent. He was a true fighter and man of principles. I admired his statuesque physical frame, his deep booming voice, and the air of authority with which he carried himself. I sensed he was overwhelmed having two daughters (my sister was born three and half years after I was). Perhaps it was because he was not familiar with the gentle subtlety of the feminine, and he was forced to learn quickly in a house that would soon have a 3:1 female-to-male ratio.

I am so grateful I have my family. In my turbulent, crazy life, in which I have to balance the needs of Sapphira and Priscilla, they have been a constant. Our family home, this place I have recently returned to for a moment of reprieve, has been a solid landing pad. Its strong brick walls are a fortress; its lilting landscape a refuge.

We were a very religious family. My parents had met as born-again Christians and were fervent in their faith and service. Going to church on a Sunday was a way of life for us and our Christian Brethren group was very strict. There are different branches of Christianity like there are different genres of music, and each branch attracts a very distinct set of people and following. Again, this is not dissimilar to music scenes and sub-cultures.

In my early years, I found the Brethren Church overall to be fun and sociable. Sunday School was a place I could be creative, but the main adult assembly meetings seemed very long and boring. I dreaded growing up and having to sit through them. As a youngster I was carefree, able to sit out in the playrooms doing arts and crafts and generally being my joyous, happy self.

The Brethren Church was a place I learnt to love music even more. There was a strong tradition of singing in both Sunday School and the main assembly meetings with the adults. My parents also bought us many sing-a-long reading books with cassette tapes, cementing my love of music. I particularly loved hearing my mother's beautiful, melodious tones soaring above everyone else in the church hall, accompanied by my father's deeper, booming bass notes. There was something about being a group of people, united in voice and resonance, that moved something deeply in all of us. It was profound and indescribable, but I felt it, young as I was. It moved me and it felt bigger than me, bigger than those of us gathered in the room, bigger than everything.

It was thanks to Sunday School that I had my first epiphany. I was about eight years old and I was invited to sing a song at the close of a theatrical play we were putting on. I chose to sing one of my personal favourites, 'In His Time', a beautiful ballad from one of my favourite Christian songbooks. I remember how nervous I was. The entire room of adults and children sat in a circle around me, a gathering of twenty or so people. As I opened my mouth to sing, I reminded myself to breathe.

Suddenly something inside me lit up. My voice, initially timid and quivering, settled into a stronger, more confident stride, and as I progressed, I began to feel something magical. It seemed as if the entire room was at a standstill, as if time itself had frozen.

There was a palpable current of energy in the air that was both breathtaking and electrifying. I was weightless, drifting in a sea of light and sound. I could not feel my body.

As I reached the final notes of the song, my voice rose in crescendo and the room burst into thunderous applause.

Momentarily I had disappeared, but the sharp staccato of applause brought me back into the room with a jolt. I focused and saw many happy, smiling faces.

It was then that I knew.

I knew I wanted to be a singer more than anything in the world.

I felt then what would become a theme in my life.

I felt The Pull.

A magnet from another dimension began tugging at my heart.

A voice I had always known began calling me. Something inside me opened up and beckoned. Without even knowing I had been asked a question, I said yes. I had found my path, my vocation – or rather it had found me.

Little did I know the turbulent journey that lay ahead of me as I began climbing my Mount Everest.

Unaware of the difficulties I would encounter on the road to self-actualisation, I took a solid first step that day. All I knew is what I felt in my heart. And from that moment, that feeling never left me.

My early years were relatively trouble free. I have a strong sense of love, interspersed with happy memories of my sister being born. I remember the joy of her falling asleep on my chest with her arms around me. It was trusting and intimate. The Brethren Church was a way of life and, like any young child, I accepted life as it was given to me without any knowledge there was even an alternative.

It was when I was around the age of eight that things began to change ...

While Sunday School presented me with the platform to sing, it was also sadly the home of less pleasurable lessons, too.

It was at Sunday School where I first learnt to feel sexual shame and inhibition. I learnt about a place called Hell and I learnt about sin. This created a deep sense of uneasiness within my soul. Knowing there was a place of eternal damnation and suffering scared the living daylights out of me. I was worried I would intrinsically be one of those people and that if I was a sinner, I would make God angry enough that he would send me to Hell forever.

While the Brethren Church was a constant theme in my childhood, there was something else that profoundly shaped my early belief systems. It is the book upon which the Brethren Church is based. To some it's known as the Scriptures; to others it's the Good Book, but to most of us it has one familiar title. It is the Bible.

A wonderfully rich source of lessons, philosophies and even erotic literature, the Bible was a book I would grow to know intimately, and more intimately than most, given that I was raised in a devoutly fervent Brethren family.

The Bible is divided into two sections: The Old Testament and the New Testament. In Sunday School we would learn the key stories from the Bible in various ways, including reading books, drawing, making paper cut-outs, listening to stories and, of course, re-enacting parts of it in the much-anticipated Sunday School Play.

Reflecting back on the premise that we are involuntarily governed by both elements of nature and nurture, I realise that something else was very evident in my personality from the beginning. The ancient Greeks called her Aphrodite. She is one of the seven female Goddess archetypes – the lover and seductress. Indeed, her presence in me was tangible. I was innocent and unaware, but my own sensual powers dwelt strongly within me, as did my ability to express that side of myself through movement.

This would prove to be a controversial theme throughout my life, but it all began at the Sunday School Play.

I was a true-born thespian, and the Sunday School Play was my first encounter with the theatre. There was a stage manager (Mrs No Nonsense), a set designer (my dad), a wardrobe department (my mum), a prop maker (my dad), a director and choreographer (Mrs No Nonsense), and promoters (my mum and dad). It didn't matter to me that we were only in a dingy church hall; this was a stage and I got to be on it. I was in heaven. (I hadn't even heard of my favourite stage light called the "follow spot" back then. Oh, the Sunday School Play I could put on now!) Nonetheless, armed with this small-scale crew, I knew I was about to make a grand entrance and I would give it my all.

Our first Sunday School production was the famous story of Daniel and the Lions' Den. I could summarise it briefly for you here but really you don't need to worry about the plot. The main thing you need to know is to look out for me on the stage. That's really all you need to know ever, so as long as you know that, we'll get on just fine!

This play would be my first experience of being what I know now to be a chorus line dancer. That's right, my first part was in fact one of the lions in Daniel's den, the ring-leader in a pack of man-eating lions. (One defenceless male was our sole target – whoever would have thought!)

The music for our play was from an American Christian music production team. They had created a slick series of songs and backing tracks, and I loved the groovy music we got to dance to as the lions. We even had leotards and little swinging tails to wear around our waists.

After a few weeks of rehearsal, the big night rolled around.

I donned my tail along with my fellow dancers and waited nervously for my chance to "go on" – a phrase I would hear many times in later years as my career progressed in show business. As the story moved forward, it came around to our part of the performance. Accompanied by my fellow lions, I made my entrance. Something similar to my first singing experience happened – I switched on!

A light bulb was switched on and I came alive. I swung my hips and wriggled my tail. I felt one with the music and the rhythm; the joy of dancing for an audience left me energised and alive. We pounced around with feline movements, our tails swooshing in time. As the number drew to a close, we fell into our final position and posed.

Like the first time I had sung, I felt a jolt of electricity. It felt great.

Unlike the first time, the applause was reserved.

We left the stage on cloud nine, the satisfying post-show adrenaline coursing through our veins. Yet there was something about this performance that was different.

Something had changed.

Later that night as we drove home in car, my father announced that there had been some disapproval among the Brothers, the men of our Christian Brethren community. He went on to explain that at future Sunday Schools there was to be no music on a sound system and that they would only use piano music instead. There would also be no dancing, no leotards and no costumes.

There was something between his words that carried a heavier meaning, a sharper disapproval. A foreboding and ominous air descended over the car. It was impenetrable, unmoving and formidable. I was frightened. I could not quite read the context of the situation. There was a cryptic message in his tone and an unspoken condemnation. I knew I had done something very, very wrong.

I panicked. I could not understand what I had done that was so bad. I was even more dumbfounded because it had felt fantastic!

A deep sense of grief set in. I lost something valuable that day, something I was too young to articulate. But it was a lesson I took into my soul. Dancing with carefree abandon was dangerous and could get me into a lot of trouble. I was worried I had upset God. I knew that he didn't like people who sinned, and I felt sure this reaction and unspoken shame from my father meant I had committed a big sin, even bigger than taking an extra cookie from the cookie tin when no one was looking at church morning tea.

Then my grief turned into anger. I was angry at Mrs No Nonsense, angry at Sunday School, and angry at myself. Deep down I was angry at God too.

That impenetrable and foreboding reaction from my father would become more and more familiar to me as I grew into adolescence. It was not long after this that I endured another traumatic scene that still dwells deep inside the recesses of my mind. I was very little and had few possessions I truly prized, but music was one thing that brought me untold, limitless joy. I had a set of favourite cassettes and records and I would listen to them over and over. But one afternoon a bizarre and disturbing incident occurred. I walked into the backyard of our home to find a bonfire burning and my father standing over it. The flames were frightening and the acrid smell even more so, singeing the hair in my nostrils, burning all the way down into the back of my throat ... As I got closer to the fire, I was shocked to see a pile of music, cassette tapes and records in my father's hands. In an eerie cleansing ritual, this fervent and protective man was burning all the non-Christian music in the house. He meant well – he wanted our home to be pure and for all our music to honour God – but I was devastated. Music was the one thing I loved and yet even my Oliver Twist record was in the pile of condemned materials. I begged and pleaded for the record not to be burnt, but my pleas fell on deaf ears. Along with Cliff Richard, Barry Manilow and many other harmless composers, my Oliver Twist record was thrown on the pile and engulfed in a ball of flames.

I lost something again that day. Something personal and private began to shut down within me. More so, I made an unconscious association with men and music: men were untrustworthy with it. This mistrust would later wreak havoc in my professional career as a singer/songwriter, as most collaboration is with males. I was scarred, and it tarnished many future interactions in the recording studio and in the music industry at large.

Sundays were not all doom and gloom, though, as some music was still allowed in my life. One favourite Sunday tradition, when we did not stay at church for the later afternoon meeting, was watching reruns of old musicals on TV. My mother was more lenient at home and loved music. It was my father who was stricter.

I adored all the musicals we watched. I loved Julie Andrews, Shirley Temple, Perry Mason, and Marilyn Monroe. Rogers and Hammerstein musicals delighted me. I revelled in the grand costumes and opulent sets, the phenomenal choreographed dance routines. I would close my eyes and picture myself on the set, one of the glamorous women. I saw myself with my eyes closed, head tilted back, being kissed by Prince Charming. I admired the tongue-in-cheek way that female sensuality was presented. It was done with such class. It was shown in the cut of a costume, the flash of a leg or an elegant gloved hand. I could drink it in for hours and I revelled in the fantasy and escapism of this bygone era. The modern-day fashions left so much to be desired in my eyes. I longed for a revival of that moment in time. The glamour and sophistication were unsurpassable.

Music ran in our family. My English grandfather loved jazz music and had been teaching himself to play piano. He died before I got to meet him. My mother was also a singer who had been in a trio act; she'd had some professional work as a young woman. She had a beautiful voice and her love of music was so strong that she had paid for her own piano lessons as a teenager out of her own pocket money.

To this day I love rifling through the hundreds of pieces of sheet music she bought. Thankfully these somehow escaped the bonfire cleansing ritual, and they truly captured a musical moment in time. They included Dusty Springfield, Carousel, and The Mamas and The Papas.

I also still had music in my life in the form of the piano, which I had started to play when I was only five years old. Because my mother always felt that she had started to learn an instrument too late in life, she was determined to provide a source of encouragement and discipline with our music lessons, the kind of support she had lacked from her own parents.

The first time I found myself sitting in front of a piano, I was entranced by the black and white keys and the sounds they made when I pushed on them with my finger. My tiny frame was dwarfed by this enormous feat of musical engineering, my small fingers barely reaching four notes apart. A sheet of music was placed in front of me, the squiggly black shapes seeming as legible as Egyptian hieroglyphics. Yet somehow, I was meant to learn what they all meant, and to create sounds from them on this gigantic wooden soundbox.

The whole process of learning an instrument was truly daunting. Miss Melancholy – my first piano teacher who always seemed to have a vacant stare to match her sparsely furnished home – was also quite scary. But my mother was determined we would learn to play piano, and thus my foray into music began.

Every day she would make sure we did our piano exercises, and it became part of family life and routine.

I frequently rebelled about the rigidity of daily practice, feigning illness regularly. But I soon learnt that there was no compromise, and secretly I was enjoying learning to play.

When I was seven years old my mother started taking me to ballet classes. The Ballet School was a delightful little studio run by Miss Ballerina. It was a tiny brick building nestled on a grassy nature strip on the main road opposite the local town hall. I liked wearing ballet slippers and leotards. Learning to dance was glorious fun, and for the first time I was put on stage outside of something involved with the Sunday School Play. It was good for my soul.

'First position, then second … lift, girls, lift!' Miss Ballerina would call to us encouragingly.

In that small, mirrored ballet studio, I would learn to plié. I learnt the various ballet positions of the feet and practised dance exercises at the barre. Yet again, I had the chance to be in a stage production and the baby showgirl in me was jigging with delight. Ballet lessons brought something else to my world. A deepening love of music was forming. This time my ears were introduced to the beauty of classic orchestral symphonies. For this introduction I owe Miss Ballerina a debt of gratitude.

Our first ballet performance was to 'Morning, Peer Gynt' by De Grieg. The haunting swell of strings stirred emotions deeply in me and I was once again swept off my feet. I heard the instruments playing in this glorious composition and it sounded as though they had their own language and were talking to each other. I wanted to understand what they were saying, and somewhere deep inside me I felt I understood, even though there were no words being exchanged. In this quiet repose and solitude, I once again felt something bigger than me and bigger than all of us. I was awestruck.

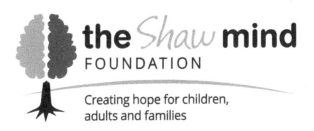

the *Shaw* mind
FOUNDATION

Creating hope for children,
adults and families

Sign up to our charity, The Shaw Mind Foundation
www.shawmindfoundation.org
and keep in touch with us; we would
love to hear from you.

*We aim to bring to an end the suffering and despair caused
by mental health issues. Our goal is to make help and support
available for every single person in society, from all walks of life.
We will never stop offering hope. These are our promises.*

Find out more

www.triggerpublishing.com

You can find us everywhere @triggerpub